Wales and Medicine

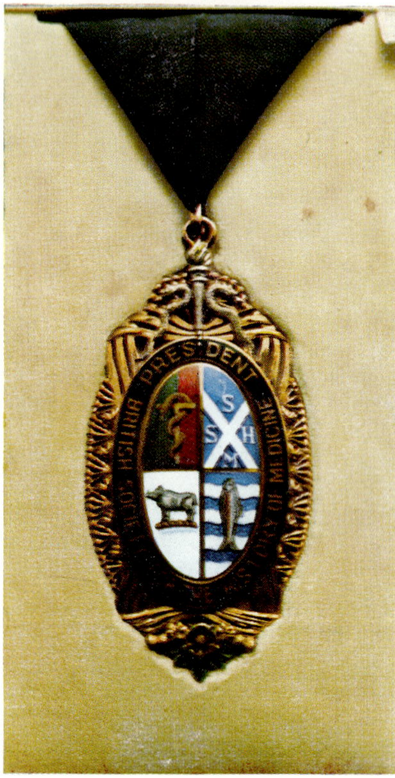
PRESIDENT
S
S H
M

Wales and Medicine

AN HISTORICAL SURVEY

FROM PAPERS GIVEN AT

THE NINTH BRITISH CONGRESS ON THE HISTORY OF MEDICINE

AT

SWANSEA & CARDIFF

4-8th SEPTEMBER, 1973

Edited by

JOHN CULE

Lecturer in the History of Medicine

Welsh National School of Medicine

Published by :

The British Society for the History of Medicine

First Impression - March 1975

SBN 85088 260 5

These papers were presented at the Ninth British Congress on the History of Medicine, which was organised by the British Society for the History of Medicine and held at the University College of Swansea and the Welsh National School of Medicine, Cardiff, between 4th and 8th September, 1973.

Printed in Wales by
J. D. LEWIS AND SONS LTD., GOMER PRESS, LLANDYSUL

CONTENTS

Contents—*Continued*

ILLUSTRATIONS

BRITISH SOCIETY FOR THE HISTORY OF MEDICINE
1973

President : Dr K. Bryn Thomas

Vice-Presidents :
Dr A. White Franklin   Dr A. Rook

Treasurer : Dr John Cule

Secretaries :
Dr D. Geraint James   Dr John Crellin

Council :

Representing Osler Club—Dr John Cule, Dr D. Geraint James, Dr Neil McIntyre.

Representing the Scottish Society for the History of Medicine—Dr A. Masson Dr H. P. Tait.

Representing the Society for the Social History of Medicine—Dr S. P. W. Chave, Dr R. G. Hodgkinson, Mr G. Wilson.

Representing the British Society for the History of Pharmacy—Dr John Crellin, Dr M. P. Earles, Dr T. D. Whittet.

Representing the Historical Section of the Royal Society of Medicine—Dr J. G. Bearn, Dr A. Rook.

Representing the Society of Apothecaries—Dr John Crellin, Dr F. N. L. Poynter, Dr G. E. W. Wolstenholme.

Representing the British Society for the History of Science—Dr W. T. Stearn.

Representing History of Medicine Society of Wales—Dr John Cule, Dr Peter Thomas.

Other members of Council—Miss Jessie Dobson, Lord Cohen of Birkenhead.

INTRODUCTION

The British Society for the History of Medicine was founded in June 1965 as a national body to represent those clubs and societies within the United Kingdom interested in the history of medicine. In order to keep this group in touch with the international scene, it now takes part in the activities of the International Society of the History of Medicine, on whose behalf it organised the 23rd International Congress of the History of Medicine, held in London, 2nd–9th September 1972. Since its foundation the Society has continued to hold biennially the national congresses on the history of medicine, originally organised by the Faculty of the History and Philosophy of Medicine and Pharmacy of the Worshipful Society of Apothecaries of London. The First British Congress on the History of Medicine and Pharmacy was held in London, 29th–30th September 1960. The Ninth British Congress was held in Wales, 4th–8th September 1973. These national and international congresses play an important part in the Society's aim to promote and encourage the study of the history of medicine.

The theme chosen for the meeting in Wales was 'Wales and Medicine'. The problems facing the medical historian in Wales are quantitatively and qualitatively different from those in England. There are fewer written Welsh sources, particularly for the earlier periods, those that exist are not easily located, and there are fewer printed diplomatic or critical texts from which the specialist can work.

For our knowledge of earlier medical practice we must rely largely on the well-known but scanty Roman accounts of the Druids, for the Druids themselves in the Celtic manner had an oral rather than a written tradition. From the sixth century onward, the Welsh language in its present form began to emerge. However, the earliest extant documents in Welsh are of the twelfth century, being copies of earlier manuscripts in Welsh of Latin now unfortunately lost. Many of the surviving manuscripts await the attention of Welsh scholars, so that medical historians may more effectively study the texts available for the mediaeval period.

From Tudor times onward, more Welshmen travelled abroad to study medicine for themselves at the English and Continental universities. Several of these doctors have left the record of their contributions to its advancement in printed books of the sixteenth century and later. Translations of Latin texts into the Welsh language continued. In more recent centuries, printed books for Welsh readers made available simple advice on health care from herbals and other English books on domestic medicine.

These sources show the story of medicine in Wales and from later biographical studies of Welsh physicians and surgeons, many of whom have published pioneer works on scientific medicine, can be seen the effect of Welshmen on the story of medicine. A great social change in medical practice was made by a Welshman who was not medically qualified. The Congress was opened by the Rt Hon. The Baroness Lee of Asheridge who spoke of ' The Contribution of Aneurin Bevan to the National Health Service '—it has unfortunately not proved possible to arrange for this personal view of her late husband to be presented for inclusion in this volume. Delegates' papers ranged widely from ' Welsh Politicians and State Medicine ', ' Disease and Medical Care in Early Wales ', ' Doctors and Literature ' and studies of the individual contributions of eminent Welsh doctors to a symposium at the Welsh National School of Medicine on the ' History of Industrial Disease '.

The Congress also included an exhibition of books and manuscripts loaned by the National Library of Wales and the Wellcome Institute of the History of Medicine, chosen to illustrate the Congress theme. Another exhibition showing ' The Evolution of Medicine in Wales ' was arranged with the help of the Welsh Folk Museum, St Fagans. Catalogues of both exhibitions have been published at the private press of the National Library of Wales.

Added flavours of Wales were given delegates, who were greeted by Geraint James at a *Noson Lawen* with Anita Williams and the Côr Gleisiaid Teifi, Llandysul ; "Under Milk Wood " was read by the Swansea Little Theatre players ; and visits were made to Brangwyn Hall, the Welsh Folk Museum and the Lower Swansea Valley Project. Major Francis Jones, Wales Herald of Arms Extraordinary was Guest of Honour at the Congress Dinner. The personal care of the staff of University College, Swansea added greatly to the success of the Congress.

The British Society gratefully acknowledges its indebtedness to Messrs E. R. Squibb and Sons Ltd for sponsoring the Congress Banquet at Cardiff Castle and for their further generous support in the publication of this volume ; to Messrs Sandoz Products Ltd for their provision of Congress transport ; to Messrs Winthrop Laboratories for their help in the production of programmes, and to The Boots Company Ltd for their donation.

It is with deep regret that we have to record the unexpected death of Dr Glyn Penrhyn Jones so shortly after he had read his paper to the Congress and before he had completed its preparation for print. His contribution to the scholarship of the history of medicine and to literature in Wales was considerable. He had clarity of style as a speaker and writer in both Welsh and English. In his company one was infected with his cheerfulness and enthusiasm. Our loss is great for he had so much more to give.

J. C.

DAVID LLOYD GEORGE
AND THE NATIONAL INSURANCE ACT OF 1911[1]

JOHN DAVIES

It is entirely fitting that the British Congress on the History of Medicine, meeting at Swansea, should devote one of its sessions to consider Lloyd George's National Insurance Act, for it was in a speech here at Swansea, sixty-five years ago this Autumn, that David Lloyd George opened the debate which was to lead to the act of 1911. On October 1, 1909 he stated at Swansea: 'There are those who through no fault of their own are unable to earn their daily bread, the aged and infirm, the broken in health, the unemployed . . . The aged we have dealt with during the present Session. We are still confronted with the more gigantic task of dealing with the rest—the sick, the infirm, the unemployed, the widows and the orphans. No country can lay any real claim to civilization that allows them to starve.'[2]

These remarks underline the basic principle behind the National Insurance Act of 1911. Its intention was not to insure the whole population against ill health but rather to insure the less affluent part of it against poverty and pauperism. It was therefore a social rather than a medical measure, aimed not so much at improving the health of the population at large but rather at providing a source of income in situations where there was no breadwinner. The turn of the century had seen the appearance of a number of studies of the incidence of poverty among the working classes and the work of Booth, Rowntree and others, soon to be amplified by the volumes of the Royal Commission on the Poor Law, indicated that between a quarter and a third of the working population of Britain lived below the poverty line and concern among social reformers was sharpened by the contrast between the desperate straits of the many and the extravagance of the few, for the Edwardian upper classes were 'the supreme hedonists of British history.'[3] The fundamental cause of poverty was seen to be an inability to obtain an income through employment and such an inability could arise, firstly through old age, secondly through sickness, thirdly through absence of work, that is involuntary unemployment, fourthly through the death of the breadwinner and fifthly through fecklessness and personal inadequacy. The aim of the major social enactments of the last Liberal governments was to provide, through the agency of the state, an income as of right for the first four categories. For the fifth category, the wilfully unemployed and unemployable, the provisions of the old and harsh poor law were deemed to be just and adequate. Nevertheless, although the old poor law survived, Liberal legislation, by recognising that people could find themselves in certain categories of poverty through no fault of their own and by providing relief as of right, created a major breach in the principle underlying the poor law, the principle which had been paramount when that law had been overhauled in 1834, that the poor were somehow morally responsible for their condition. Of all the bars to employment which caused pauperism, the most important was old age and this was dealt with in the old age pension legislation of 1908. The logical next step was to legislate for the provision of income for those threatened by pauperism through sickness, unemployment or the death of the breadwinner and this was the intention of the legislation of 1911. In no sense did the Liberals seek to create a comprehensive health service, nor did they seek to build a coherent edifice inspired by a philosophical belief in the virtues of collective control. The National Insurance Act was the product of facts not of theories and concerned itself with sickness mainly as a cause of pauperism. The scheme did not originally include treatment of illness and at no time was there any intention of insuring housewives for, as a report of 1910 put it, 'as long as the husband is able to work, adequate provision will be made for the needs of the family, irrespective of the wife's health, whereas, when the husband's health fails, there is no one to earn the wages'.[4]

Before examining Lloyd George's role in the establishment of national insurance, it may be useful to give some account of the act itself. It was introduced into the Commons on 4th March 1911 and, after a long struggle and many amendments, received royal assent on the 6th November. The act was divided into two parts: the second dealing with unemployment and the first, with which we are now concerned, dealing with insurance against sickness. This specified that all manual workers and all other workers earning less than £160 a year were obliged to insure themselves at the rate of fourpence per week (threepence for women) to which sum the employer added threepence and the state twopence. Stamps to this value, bought at the post office, were stuck on a card which was then taken by the insured to an approved society of his choice, which administered the scheme on behalf of the government. In return, if the insured were incapacitated by illness, the society would pay him ten shillings a week for the first twenty-six weeks (7s. 6d. for women) and five shillings disability benefit thereafter and would also pay for medical attention and drugs. In addition, a thirty shillings maternity benefit was to be paid, one and a half million pounds was to be raised for the building of sanatoria for the treatment of tuberculosis and grants were to be made for research, making possible the establishment of the Medical Research Council. Payments were to begin in July 1912 and benefits in January 1913.

Such a scheme, which proposed compulsorily to insure up to fifteen million people and directly affecting, through their families, a total of thirty nine million could not, of course be created in a vacuum. Such a major enactment was possible in 1911 because of the developments and the experience of the preceeding years, but equally, the full realisation of Lloyd George's vision was not possible because in those preceeding years attitudes, institutions and vested interests had arisen whose hostility to a more comprehensive scheme could not be overcome. On the credit side was the development of the organs of the state. National insurance needed an army of officials and a tradition of bureaucratic service which was almost wholly absent in early Victorian Britain but which had developed by the early twentieth century. Estimating the demands that would be made upon the service necessitated an array of actuarial skills which had been evolved by the friendly societies and the insurance companies in the course of the nineteenth century. The efficient running of the service needed men experienced in the collecting of information and the handling of statistics, again skills which had been acquired through the growth of a more complex state structure. The importance of reliable statistics was highlighted when old age pensions at 70 were introduced in Ireland in 1909. Regular registrations of births had not begun there until 1865 and few aged Irishmen had any documentary proof of their age. A singularly large number claimed that their parents had told them they had been born in the year of the ' big wind ', which turned out to be 1839 and thus conveniently qualified them for pensions. The 1911 census showed that there was in Ireland a total of 191,720 people over 70 ; 201,783 Irish pensioners had, however, in that year received pensions.[5]

On the debit side, the chief obstacle Lloyd George faced in seeking a more thoroughgoing scheme with a fuller recognition of state obligation, was the laissez-faire tradition which was disturbed by an extension of state interference. There is evidence to suggest that Lloyd George wished to see such a fuller recognition,[6] but he was aware that doctrinaire anti-collectivism and Gladstonian traditions of retrenchment and orthodox finance were still deeply rooted in the Liberal party. Leading members of the cabinet lacked enthusiasm for social reform and to many of the more traditional Liberals, Lloyd George's zeal was an embarrassment. There was, of course, a tradition of state interference in Britain in the interests of health, beginning with the sanitary agitation of the mid-nineteenth century. There was a basic difference, however, between the course of action advocated by health reformers in the mid-nineteenth century and that advocated by the reformers of the early twentieth, a difference symbolised, perhaps, by the contrast between the dread disease of the 1850's, and the dread disease of the 1910's. It was cholera which terrified in the 1850's and it could be countered not by making elaborate provision for the patient but by providing a cleaner environment. Thus the key issue then was public health rather than individual health and the key figure was the sanitary inspector rather than the doctor, and the sanitary agitation was so effective that it could be claimed that the British genius consisted of an infinite capacity for making drains. It was tuberculosis which terrified in the 1910's and while that was also, in a sense, a disease of the environment, it could only be countered by skilled and sustained nursing at the individual level. Eradicating tuberculosis, particularly among those who could not afford to pay for their own treatment, demanded a far more radical role for the state than had the eradication of cholera. Lloyd George understood the logic of the situation but a fuller recognition of state obligation would have been resisted by his colleagues and rather than jeopardise everything, he had to be content with something less than a full realisation of his vision.

A further factor preventing the establishment of a coherent health service was the poor law with its deterrent traditions, its assumption that destitution was the prerequisite of aid and the fear and hatred felt towards it by the poorer sections of community. In 1909 the Minority Report of the Royal Commission on the Poor Law recommended its abolition and the placing of wide ranging social services under local authorities. Such radical action was, however, not to the taste of the minister responsible for its operation, John Burns, the President of the Local Government Board and he even refused to implement the milder suggestions of the Majority Report. As there was no hope of abolishing the poor law, the relationship between it and national insurance was a delicate matter. To link the two would be to sacrifice everything, for insurance would thereby have been damned in the eyes of those it was intended to help. Thus national insurance was not a replacement of the poor law but rather a by-passing of it. Lloyd George was determined to keep the two wholly separate and his scorn for Burns was such that he gave the Local Government Board no role in his scheme. National insurance was to be controlled by Insurance Commissioners directly answerable to the Treasury. As a result, responsibility for health was fragmented between the Local Government Board, the Insurance Commissioners and, for school children, the Board of Education, creating, perhaps inevitably, a cumbersome and bureaucratic structure.

Hatred and fear of the poor law had led the British working classes to create or to support alternative institutions in the hope of remaining outside its grasp. Chief among these were the friendly societies such as the Odd fellows and the Ivorites and the industrial insurance companies such as the Prudential and the Pearl. By the early twentieth century over six million people had ensured against sickness with the friendly societies, an imposing number, but the fact that this figure included only half, and the wealthier half, of wage earners, coupled with the financial instability of a number of the societies, was one of the strongest arguments in favour of compulsory state insurance. Some 42 million insurance policies for funeral benefit were in existence in 1911.[7] This was the most popular insurance of all, for at 1d or 2d a week a man could be insured against the final humiliation of a pauper burial. Investigators into poverty collected much evidence of the pride shown by working class widows in their ability to bury their husbands with dignity : 'I put him away splendid' said one; 'I buried him with ham ' said another.[8] The creation of national insurance meant that the state was appropriating functions fulfilled, albeit imperfectly, by other institutions and early in the progress of his bill Lloyd George realised that he would have to come to some accommodation with these institutions. To the friendly societies he was well disposed and most of them were appointed approved societies to implement the scheme with the right, originally, directly to employ the doctors who provided medical attention to the insured. Industrial insurance companies he disliked but could not ignore. The Prudential Company was the largest shareholder of Bank of England stocks and the companies between them employed 70,000 full-time agents who were in weekly contact with working class homes—an army far greater than that of any political party and one which any politician would hesitate to alienate.[9] The companies were determined that nothing should interfere with their lucrative death insurance and thus stubbornly resisted Lloyd George's scheme for widows' and orphans' pensions. Their opposition was successful and such pensions did not feature in the Act thus removing one category of potential pauperism from the hope of succour by the state. They also insisted on becoming approved societies on a par with the friendly societies, a concession which caused much disillusion to the more radical advocates of national insurance.

More serious was the opposition of the doctors. They feared that the extension of insurance would rob them of lucrative, private, fee-paying patients, that they would become tied servants of the friendly societies, that patients would have no free choice of doctor, that payment would be insufficient and that the state would interfere in the private relationship between patient and doctor. The British Medical Association leadership took up an intransigent position on the matter and threatened to wreck the whole scheme. Lloyd George, who considered doctors the most touchy and suspicious of all professional groups (although as a member of the legal profession himself he should have known better) brought all his talents to bear in dealing with them. While conceding most of their demands, he skilfully divided the leadership from the rank and file. ' It is difficult to ascertain the true feelings of doctors as a whole on any proposal affecting them ' he stated, ' since a deputation of doctors is always a deputation of swell doctors ; it is impossible to get a deputation of poor doctors or of slum doctors '.[10] In his meetings with the B.M.A. he was at his most brilliantly persuasive and he said of one such meeting that there had been 'nothing like it since Daniel entered the lion's den'.[11] In the event the National Insurance Act became the general practitioner's charter: only one fifth of all general practitioners stayed outside the scheme and doctors in poorer areas saw their income increased and their prestige enhanced.[12]

In the country at large in 1911, National insurance was far from popular. Old age pensions were widely acclaimed; perhaps the best known tribute is that in Flora Thompson's autobiographical study *Lark Rise* where she quotes rural cottagers in Oxfordshire as saying "'God bless that Lord George' (for they could not believe one so powerful and munificent could be a plain 'Mr')."[13] National insurance, however, was bitterly attacked and there can be little doubt that had a general election been held in 1911 the government, because of Lloyd George's activities, would have been heavily defeated.[14] Workers disliked the element of compulsion in the contributions; socialists and Fabians were tireless in pointing out the contradictions and inadequacies of the measure;[15] insurance agents were poisoning minds against it on the door-steps; the Northcliffe press ran a scurrilous campaign against Lloyd George and all his works and the Tories, smarting under their defeat over the budget and the House of Lords found the unpopularity of the act a useful stick with which to beat the government. Perhaps the oddest opposition came from society ladies and their maids who revolted at the idea of sticking stamps in a book at the behest of Lloyd George. At the end of November a mammoth protest rally was held at the Albert Hall, where the stage was graced by both the Dowager Countess Desart and her maid. Before the meeting began martial airs were played but when the organist played Men of Harlech, the hissing was so intense that Rule Britannia had rapidly to be substituted.[16]

In the face of such varied opposition and such deep-seated vested interests, it was inevitable that the National Insurance Act was far from perfect. It had been hurriedly carried through and its implementers faced major difficulties in its early months; state provision for health was fragmented and too many concessions had been made to the industrial insurance companies; widows and orphans had been left without coverage and no adequate provision had been made for hospitals.

Yet, the fact remains that the achievement was staggering. The measure affected thirty nine million people, a far higher proportion than was covered by Bismarck's much vaunted scheme in Germany.[17] The saving in lives, in suffering, in humiliation was incalculable and the reformers of the 1940's inherited a stable framework of central and local organisation in the field of health capable of sustaining a more complex and comprehensive service.

This was Lloyd George's achievement for, despite the dedicated assistance of some of his government colleagues, particularly C. F. Masterman at the Home Office and Winston Churchill and of tireless civil servants such as W. J. Braithwaite and Robert Morant, it is impossible to believe that such a wide-ranging scheme could have been conceived and carried through without him. No active cabinet minister before Lloyd George had had his intuitive understanding of working class needs or had 'known the life of the people so well'.[18] It was he who conciliated the doctors and it was he, in the dark days of November 1911, when Asquith seemed prepared to jettison the whole project, who pushed it through by sheer endurance and heroic demagogy. And when insurance was at its most unpopular, it was he who coined the most telling slogan of all: 'ninepence for fourpence'. (He did so, incidentally, at a meeting at Whitefield's Tabernacle; it was odd to choose so Calvinist a place in which to present anything as a lottery in which everyone wins prizes).

Perhaps the last word should be left to Winston Churchill, Lloyd George's faithful lieutenant in the last Liberal Governments, who, in his tribute in the House of Commons in March 1945 declared:

> 'It was Lloyd George who launched the Liberal and Radical forces of this country effectively into the broad stream of social betterment and social security along which all modern parties now steer . . . Most people are now unconscious of how much their lives have been shaped by the laws for which Lloyd George was responsible. Health insurance and old age pensions were the first large-scale state conscious efforts to set a balustrade along the crowded causeway of the people's life and, without pulling down the structures of society, to fasten a lid over the abyss into which vast numbers used to fall'[19].

NOTES

1 The authoritative account of the measure is B. B. Gilbert, *The Evolution of National Insurance in Great Britain* (Joseph, London, 1966). There are accounts of the progress of the bill through parliament in É. Halévy, *The History of the English People in the Nineteenth Century*, vol. VI, *The Rule of Democracy*, 1905–1914 (first paperback edition, Benn, London, 1961) pp. 350–68 and in P. Rowland, *The Last Liberal Governments*, vol. 2, *Unfinished Business*, 1911–14. (Barrie & Jenkins, London, 1971) pp. 32–35, 80–86. The act is discussed within the broad context of social reform in M. Bruce, *The Coming of the Welfare State* (Batsford, London, 1961) and within the context of Liberal ideology in H. V. Emy, *Liberals, radicals and Social Politics*, 1892–1914 (Cambridge University Press, London, 1973).

2 D. Lloyd George, *Better Times* (Hodder & Stoughton, London, 1910) p.53.

3 M. Bruce, *op.cit.*, p. 135.

4 B. B. Gilbert, *op.cit.*, p. 315.

5 *Ibid., pp.* 227–28.

6 See M. Bruce, *op.cit.*, p. 174. Compare T. Jones, *Lloyd George* (Oxford University Press, London, 1951) pp. 39–40.

7 M. Bruce, *op.cit.*, p. 97. Compare B. B. Gilbert, *op.cit.*, p. 319.

8 *Ibid.*, p. 321n.

9 *Ibid.*, pp. 319–20.

10 *Ibid.*, p. 363.

11 M. Bruce., *op.cit* p. 118.

12 B. B. Gilbert, *op.cit.*, pp. 437–41.

13 F. Thompson, *Lark Rise to Candleford* (Oxford University Press, London, 1945) p. 86.

14 See P. Rowland, *op.cit.*, vol. II, p. 80 ; T. Jones, *op.cit.*, pp. 40–41 ; H. V. Emy, *op.cit.*, p. 255 and B. B. Gilbert, *op.cit.*, pp. 394–95.

15 For a socialist attack upon the National Insurance Act see G. D. H. Cole and R. Postgate, *The Common People* (Paperback edition, Methuen, London 1961) pp. 469–70. A Fabian viewpoint is given in Beatrice Webb, *Our Partnership*, ed. by B. Drake and M. I. Cole (Longmans, London, 1948) pp. 468, 473–74, 477–79. The imposition of burdens, not upon the citizens as a whole, but upon the low paid and ' the vulgar fellow working with his hands ' aroused the ire of Hilaire Belloc (*The servile state*, Foulis, London, 1912, pp. 164–65).

16 B. B. Gilbert, *op.cit.*, p. 396.

17 For a comparison of the two schemes, see É. Halévy, *op.cit.*, pp. 352–54.

18 *Parliamentary debates*, (Hansard) (H.M.S.O., London 1945), fifth series, vol. 409, p. 1378.

19 *Ibid.* Compare W. S. Churchill, *Liberalism and the Social Problem* (Hodder and Stoughton, London, 1909) p. 82.

SOME EARLY WELSH CONTRIBUTORS TO AMERICAN MEDICINE
THE FAMILY OF JONES

K. BRYN THOMAS

When setting off on this quest for the Welsh founders of American medicine I only vaguely realised the problems of sources and identification which would raise their heads during my search, particularly as it has been confined to this side of the Atlantic ; in few cases is it possible to identify families and origins in Wales.

Only by their names shall you know them and their names, if not legion, are certainly multiplicated !

Glenn's *Welsh Founders of Pennsylvania* contains a list of some of the founders in which there are fifty Joneses, some of whom were also called John, or changed their name from Lloyd, and five of whom were Cadwalader Jones (or John) with seven Thomases, five Roberts and four Evan Joneses. Of these, only one was a medical man, Edward Jones, whom we shall note later. The reasons for such multiplicity are well known and do not concern us here ; one may merely mention that fixed surnames were not common in Wales until the early seventeen hundreds.

Perusal of the *American Dictionary of Biography* or the *Surgeon-General's Catalogue,* both of which contain many Evanses, Williamses and Joneses, does not reveal any early works by the pioneers. Then one realises that these men hardly found the time or opportunity to go into print, even if they could find a printer. Thus seventeenth or early eighteenth century records are few. It was not until the cities became established, with their more stable populations, that the wealthier members began to send their sons to Europe for their education ; and not till the mid-eighteenth century that second or third generation Americans, returning to their native lands in the West, began the great awakening of American medicine.

When one finds that the only American medical treatise of the seventeenth century was that of Thomas Thacher on *Small Pocks or Measles* (Boston, 1677) it is apparent that minute searching is required to track down any emigrant of the early colonial days who took to the practice of medicine. This work has been done by diligent scholars of the past and I can present no new primary evidence.

Few of the early medical men were qualified physicians, though some were clergy who had undergone a training in medicine prior to emigrating, as a precaution in case of removal from their beneficiaries. Such men were William Brewster (1560?-1644), leader in the plan for emigration, and Edward Winslow (1595-1655), one of the Pilgrim Fathers. Of these original names, none appears as a Welshman, though the captain of the *Mayflower* was Christopher Joanes. The names are known of twenty-six graduates of Harvard College before 1700, who practised medicine in New England. None of these came of Welsh stock, so far as is apparent.

Medicine was learned, as in England, by apprenticeship. In many instances a family line of doctors was set up, as in the case of the Clark family, founded by John Clark (1598-1664) who went to Boston in about 1638 : the seventh John Clark proceeded M.D. from Havard in 1802, the only one of the long line of over 150 years to receive a degree.

Oliver Wendell Holmes in *Medical Essays,* 1883, gave a fascinating account of an imaginary visit to the patient of a preacher-physician, one Giles Firmin, who was a historical figure, and who had been the first American to teach anatomy from the cadaver, about 1640. Holmes makes Firmin ride with his apprentice, Luke, to see a patient with colic. The lad thinks the man may die, but Firmin says ' 'tis but a dry belly ache . . . he hath not the pulse of them with fevers . . . we will steep certain comforting herbs and put them in a bag and lay them on his belly. Likewise he shall have my cordial julep with a portion of this confection which hath juice of poppy in it and is a great stayer of anguish.' We shall hear again of the use of opium in dry belly ache, when we meet Thomas Cadwalader.

Similarly, Garrison noted the importance of the apprentice system in training the young doctor, mentioning also another important feature of early colonial medicine.

> Under primitive frontier conditions the mediaeval antagonism between physicians and surgeons soon disappears, for the necessary

and sufficient reason that, while midwifery was in the hands of women, the open country or backwoods doctor was liable to be called on in any emergency. Thrown upon his own resources he soon learned to enlarge such native skill as he had in bone-setting, treatment of arrow and gun-shot wounds or reducing hernias, and so became a bit of a surgeon.

This was the setting in which early colonial doctors lived and practised.

THE WELSHMEN

Study of the *American Dictionary of Biography* or the *Surgeon-General's Catalogue* is a hit and miss business. Which Jones shall we select? Edward, of Philadelphia, who wrote on pneumonia in 1796, John, the surgeon of New York and Philadelphia, or Samuel of the hydrocoele, 1797. Of the Williamses, John wrote of the unlawfulness of inoculation in 1721, and on yellow fever in 1750, while Nathanael described his method of inoculation in 1752. In any case, it is not safe to assume that these gentlemen all came from Welsh families in spite of their names, in the absence of other evidence. There is for example, James Lloyd (1726-1810) who was for fifty years one of the great New England physicians, bearing an ancient and famous Cymric name. His grandfather had emigrated from Bristol and we can trace no direct Welsh connection. For similar reasons, it is not allowable to discuss Samuel Powel Griffitts, M.D. (1759-1826) son of William Griffitts and Abigail Powell, surely a Welsh combination; or Dr Cadwalader Evans, physician to the Pennsylvania Hospital, who was captured by pirates in the Caribbean on his way to Edinburgh, and who as a student published a note on a case of convulsions in a girl of 14, which was cured after ten years, by electricity 'given by the scientific hands of Dr Franklin.'

I do not propose to do other than mention here the famous name of Dr John Morgan, (1735-1789), about whom much has been written, including Whitfield Bell's fine biography. Pupil of the Hunters, co-founder with Shippen of the Philadelphia Medical School, controversial Director General of Washington's army, Morgan's stormy career ended in a sad old age. His family is believed to have come from Glamorgan.

DR THOMAS WYNNE, 1627-1692

A family tree of north Walian emigrant doctors shows Dr Thomas Wynne (1627-1692) of Bron Vadog in the parish of Ysceifiog, near Caerwys, Flintshire, as the American progenitor. He emigrated with William Penn himself, in September 1682 on the ship *Welcome*. He was an early and staunch member of the Society of Friends, suffering imprisonment for his beliefs. In 1677 Wynne wrote a pamphlet, partly in Welsh, entitled *The Antiquity of the Quakers proved out of the Scriptures of Truth, Published in Love to the Papists, Protestants, Presbyterians, Independents and Anabaptists, with a Salutation of pure love to all the Tender-Hearted Welshmen. But more especially to Flintshire, Denbighshire, Caernarvonshire and Anglesea. By their Countryman and friend, Thomas Wynne, Printed in the Year* 1677.

This pamphlet was answered by a William Jones, in a booklet containing what Glenn calls a ' finely etched portrait of Thomas Wynne tempted by the Devil.' It has not been possible to trace a copy.

Quaker families in Wales had suffered particularly severe persecution and were ready to seek a land offering peace and independence, where they might also preserve their language and ancient customs. So Thomas Wynne was sent as one of a committee of twelve to meet William Penn in London. Penn's grant of land was made by the king on 5 March 1681, who was sympathetic to their cause. With John ap John of Llangollen, Wynne took up a patent dated 15 September 1681, for 5,000 acres in Pennsylvania, for £100 and a quit-rent. It is said too that he built one of the first brick houses in Philadelphia. Wynne died there in 1692 and is described in his will as ' practitioner in physic.'

We know little of his practice, but another pamphlet of his, of 1679, that is before he left Wales, gives an interesting insight into his early medical career.

' My genious from a child ' wrote Wynne ' did lead me to surgery, insomuch that before I was ten years old, I several times over-ran my school and home when I heard of anyone's being wounded or hurt and used all my endeavours to see Fractures and Dislocations reduced and wounds dressed . . . my parents thought they had lost me for which I underwent severe correction. My Father died before I was eleaven years old and my Mother [was] not able to produce so great a sum as to set me to chyrurgery . . . until I became acquainted with an honest friend, and good artist in Chyrurgery whose name was Richard Moore of Salop, who seeing my forwardness to Chyrurgery, did further me in it, and brought me to Disections in Salop ; the Anatomists being men of known worth in that Practice, whose names are Dr. Needham and Dr. Hollins . . . I being then expert in Drills and Handy in Knife and Lancet . . . I set on making a Skeleton of a man's bones, which I only with the assistance of Richard Moore performed to their content, at which time they thought me fit to be Licensed the practice of Chyrurgery, and this is near 20 years ago and soon after I being taken a Prisoner to Denbigh, where I remained a prisoner for near six years for the Testimony of Jesus, I then betook myself wholly to the practice of Chyrurgery.'

Walter Needham, *c* 1631-1691, was a comparative anatomist, author of *De Formatu Foetu,* 1667.

DR EDWARD JONES, 1645-1737

Thomas Wynne's eldest child Mary married Dr Edward Jones (1645-1737) of Bala, in 1676, six years before they emigrated with two small children. They sailed from Liverpool in the *Lion*, Captain Compton, and arrived in Philadelphia in August 1682, shortly before Thomas Wynne. Thus in 1682, Wynne, Edward Jones and a Dr Griffith Owen (a Welsh name indeed though he came from Lancashire) all members of the Society of Friends, were the first physicians to go to Pennsylvania. In company with sixteen other persons, all from the Bala district, Edward Jones had acquired 5,000 acres of land from William Penn at a cost of £100. His own share was 312½ acres for £6.5.0. Within two weeks of arrival he wrote describing the arrangements of the lots, 'the end of each lot will be on a river as large or larger than the Dye (Dee) at Bala, it is called Skool Kill River' (i.e. Schuylkill). Edward Jones played a leading part in setting up the new *Welsh Tract*, naming it Merion, after their native county in Wales. We know little of his medical activities, but he was a prominent citizen in rapidly expanding Philadelphia, and a successful agriculturalist. He died at Merion in 1727 at the age of ninety-two.

Edward Jones and Mary Wynne had eight children. The eldest Martha, born in Wales, married John Cadwalader (1677-1733) in Philadelphia in 1699. Their son Thomas was a physician of whom more will be told. The fifth child of Edward and Mary Jones, Evan, was apprenticed in medicine to his father and became father of the famous surgeon John Jones. Thus Thomas Cadwalader and John Jones were first cousins, though twenty years separated them in age. Each made important contributions to the medical life of New England.

THOMAS CADWALADER, 1708-1779

Thomas Cadwalader grandson of Edward Jones, was born in Philadelphia in 1708. The city was then an expanding and increasingly important centre, with a population of some 10,000 souls. Thomas served his medical apprenticeship under his uncle Dr Evan Jones and under Dr John Kearsley, a notable English emigrant physician.

In his early twenties, Cadwalader proceeded to England to study under William Cheselden, then the doyen of English surgery. It is a comment upon the rising prosperity of Philadelphia that it could afford to send its students for the European tour. Thomas Cadwalader was one of the earliest young physicians to do so. Returning to Philadelphia in 1730 with much training, but with no medical degree he went into practice and rapidly began to make a name. In this same year he was responsible for the production of anatomical preparations for the elder Dr William Shippen, and he filled a great local need by giving a series of dissections for students. At the age of twenty-five, he assisted Benjamin Franklin (1706-1790) in the foundation of the Philadelphia Library and was its director from 1731-1739. He was a pioneer of inoculation against smallpox, at that time still a controversial matter, though Zabdiel Boylston (1679-1766) had introduced it into Boston in 1721 ; Cadwalader's advocacy provided an important impetus for the method in Philadelphia, though he published nothing on the subject.

In 1738 Cadwalader married Hannah Lambert, daughter of a wealthy landowner in Trenton, New Jersey, and retired to Trenton, where he appears only occasionally to have used his medical knowledge. In 1751 we find him again in Philadelphia taking an active part in the founding of the Pennsylvania Hospital. He was not officially appointed to the staff, but to within two years of his death in 1779, he assisted in 'Consultations on extraordinary Cases', to quote the minute of the Board of Managers.

Like so many other Colonial professional men, Cadwalader was a staunch patriot of his native land, developing strong feelings against the British government and objecting violently to the *Stamp Acts* which were so provocative a factor in the onset of the Revolutionary War. His two sons General John and Colonel Lambert Cadwalader played active parts in the conduct of the War. Dr Cadwalader however maintained his professional impartiality, earning the gratitude of General Prescott, later Governor of Canada, for treating him while a prisoner of war, and for reporting on the insanitary conditions of the wartime gaol. Prescott later secured the release of Colonel Lambert Cadwalader, who in turn had been captured by the British.

Cadwalader made two interesting medical observations, both contained in his book entitled *An Essay on the West-India dry-gripes with the method of preventing that cruel distemper , to which is added an extraordinary case in physick.* Philadelphia. 1745. The publisher was Benjamin Franklin. This is sometimes referred to as An *Essay on the Iliac Passion.* The autograph manuscript is in the historical collection of the College of Physicians of Philadelphia, but of the work itself few copies are extant. The ' dry-gripes ' was an expressive term used to describe the colic produced by lead poisoning, though Cadwalader did not recognise this cause. He described in graphic detail the paralysis constipation and abdominal pain, and the encephalopathy associated with lead-poisoning.

> The European physicians give an account of a disease similar to the Dry-Gripes, . . . attended with excessive gripping pains in the pit of the stomach and bowels . . . there is a sensation as if the Bowels were drawn together by Ropes.

His notions of the pathology are shown by this passage :

> The Alcaline Acrimony impacted on the Stomach and intestines is so great in many cases as to communicate its malign influence to the whole nervous system causing violent convulsions which are very dangerous symptoms . . . But if the excessive Pain continues any considerable time, the Peristaltic Motion of the intestines become inverted, and the *Iliac Passion* ensues. This sore malady usually degenerates into the Palsy and a deprivation of all sort of Motion in the Hands and Feet.

He quoted the case of a man of forty with dry-gripes treated at a London Hospital with 18oz of liquid mercury. At the autopsy a week later 14oz of ' quicksilver ' were found in the stomach, and Cadwalader suggested that this might be an improper method of treatment ! He advised also against the use of ' strong punch ' and (perhaps unnecessarily in such a condition) against general activities such as immoderate exercise and ' profuse venery.' His own treatment sensibly recommended opium with mild cathartics in place of the usual purging and mercury. In spite of his lack of knowledge of the cause, Cadwalader mentioned that colic may be caused by the fumes of whitelead, a notable reference. It is also to be remarked that Benjamin Franklin considered the book worthy of publication, and that Franklin himself was later to show (in 1786) that the disease was the result of the habitual drinking of Jamaica rum distilled through leaden pipes. An interesting parallel may be drawn between this history of the disease in America and the description of Devonshire colic by John Huxham in 1739 (six years before Cadwalader), and the discovery of its connection with lead in cider vats by Sir George Baker in 1767, some twenty years before Franklin's similar finding.

Cadwalader's ' extraordinary case in physic ' to quote his title, was that of a woman who died from osteomalacia. Cadwalader's autopsy in 1742, was not only one of the earliest such examinations to be reported in America, but was also the first to be made on the disease, though it had been described in 1705 by Jean-Louis Petit of Paris. The patient was a forty year old woman whose ' Bones in her legs and arms felt somewhat soft to the touch and were so pliable as to be bent into a curve.' At autopsy, Cadwalader found the outer laminae of the bones soft and perfectly membranous, about ' the thickness of the peritonaeum : and containing (instead of a bony substance) a fluid of the consistency of honey when thick and of a reddish colour.' ' Quaere ? whether a corrosive acid state of the fluids might not have been the cause of this uncommon dissolution of the bones ? Quaere ? whether an alkaline regimen, timely pursued, would not have been the most likely method to have succeeded in this poor woman's case ? ' Such queries on the pathology are interesting, if almost meaningless today. It was nearly two hundred years before the causes of *ossies mollitum* were elucidated ; the part played by vitamin D was demonstrated in 1929 by J. P. Maxwell (1871-1961).

JOHN JONES, 1729-1791

The other medical grandson of Edward Jones was born in Jamaica, Long Island, N.Y. His father Evan had studied with his grandfather, Edward Jones, and had then moved to New York where he introduced inoculation against small-pox. John Jones returned to Philadelphia for apprenticeship to his cousin, Thomas Cadwalader. Like him, Jones too took the grand tour at the age of twenty, coming to England to attend the lectures of William Hunter where he would have met John Hunter, of his own age, employed at the dissection table. Jones also worked at St Bartholomew's Hospital under Percival Pott, and went on to Paris to sit at the feet of Jean-Louis Petit, leading French surgeon, and Henri Francois le Dran, whose knowledge and skill as a lithotomist must have influenced the young man's future work. In 1751, Jones received a medical doctorate at Rheims for a thesis entitled *Observations on Wounds*, later to be published in New York. These American and other student tourists of the eighteenth century acquired a full and varied medical education ; but they had to go in search of it and they needed stamina, the will to learn—and money. We find no direct evidence that John Jones possessed these gifts,—the evidence lies in his journeys and in his subsequent eminent career.

Back in New York in the 1750's Jones soon acquired an extensive practice, particularly in lithotomy. At this time, Cheselden's lateral approach to the bladder was the accepted method for the removal of stone, and it is stated that Jones (like Cheselden) would perform the operation successfully in three minutes. Garrison says that he was remembered in the will of Benjamin Franklin for performing the operation. In fact, Jones was a personal friend and physician of both George Washington and Franklin whom he attended in his last illness, of which he published an account in the *Pennsylvania Gazette*-21 April 1770. In 1755 Jones volunteered as a surgeon in the French-Indian War in Canada. His previous interest in wounds, and his experiences as a military surgeon, were later to culminate in a famous book, *Plain Concise Practical Remarks on the Treatment of Wounds and Fractures, to which is added an appendix on Camp and Military Hospitals, principally designed for the use of young military and naval surgeons in North America.* Philadelphia. 1776. It is remarkable that America waited so long for a medical book by one of her own sons, yet this was indeed the first. Billings remarks that it is simply a compilation from Pott and others containing but one original observation. This unique precedent has not been discovered, but the appendix is notable for its *Hints concerning military hospitals* in which the accent is on fresh air, diet and cleanliness, including clean and warm bedding.

In 1776 also the book was re-issued bound with van Swieten's *Diseases incident to Armies*, translated by Jones himself: the combination proved both popular and valuable, the van Swieten addition adding greatly to the original. A third edition appeared in 1795, edited by James Meare M.D. as *Surgical Works of the late John Jones*, with a biography of Jones written by Meare.

In 1768, Jones returned to London, believing that the air in the *great wen* relieved his asthma. He again attended the lectures of William Hunter and Pott and must have known Fothergill. He raised funds for the foundation of New York's first hospital, and returning to his practice, was driven thence when New York was captured by the British. He moved to Philadelphia, which suited his health, to set up once again in practice ; at this time, too he played an important part in organising the medical department of the continental army and was appointed to the Pennsylvania Hospital. He was a first vice-president of the College of Physicians of Pennsylvania on its foundation in 1787, and contributed a paper *On Anthrax*, published posthumously in the first volume of its *Transactions* in 1793.

Miss Dobson in a personal communication, draws attention to two eponyms : *Jones's Position*—acute flexion of the fore-arm for the treatment of fracture of the medial condyle of the humerus ; *Jones's splint* for fracture of the nasal bones.

John Jones was a staunch republican ; Meare quoted his remark that he considered titles as a ' pagentry of Coxcombs '. His extant letters to the lawyer James Duane (1733-1797) of New York, show him also to have been a ' conservative patriot ' to borrow Steven Charles' phrase, deeply concerned with the cause of independence, but chiefly anxious that it should be obtained without bloodshed.

John Jones died in Philadelphia on 22 June, 1791.

JOHN JONES AND THE NEW YORK MEDICAL SCHOOL AND HOSPITAL

On 4 August 1767, five medical men of New York, Samuel Clossy, Peter Middleton, John Jones, James Smith and Samuel Bard, wrote a letter to the governors of King's College, later to become Columbia College and University, which had been founded some twelve years earlier. They suggested the foundation of a school of physic with five professorships, one for each of them, of which that in the *Theory of Chirurgery* should be held by Jones. The Governors of King's College agreed and the School of Physic commenced its lectures in November 1767, the five original signatories being appointed to the Chairs :-

Samuel Closey, M.D.	—	anatomy
Peter Middleton, M.D.	—	theory of physic
John Jones, M.D.	—	chirurgery
James Smith, M.D.	—	chymistry and materia medica
Samuel Bard, M.D.	—	practice of physic.

John Tennent was added as professor of midwifery.

All these were names well-known in New York medical circles. In particular, Samuel Bard, (1742-1821), brought up to medicine by his astute physician father, John Bard, had gone to London in 1762, armed with a letter from John Jones to Fothergill. In London and Edinburgh Bard was a fellow student with John Morgan, and these two had discussed their mutual ambitions for the establishment of a medical school in America on the lines of the Edinburgh School. Samuel Bard wrote to his father in December 1762 'I wish with all my heart . . . I might assist in founding the first medical college in America . . . if such a thing was undertaken it ought to be in conjunction with [King's] College.'

So it turned out, though the College of Physic founded in 1768 by Jones and Bard and their confreres was not the first in the States. That honour went to the Medical School of Philadelphia, founded, not without strife, by John Morgan and William Shippen in 1765. Stookey however, remarks that the Philadelphia Medical School had opened with only two professors 'and cannot be said to have met the requirements of a Medical School. It would appear that the dis tinction of having the first medical school with a complete faculty of six professors offering courses in all subjects then taught as a part of a collegiate undertaking, belongs to King's College.' However this may be, the two earliest schools of medicine in America each had a founding Welshman. Unfortunately the New York medical school failed to survive the Revolution, though resurrected in 1792 as the Medical Faculty of Columbia College.

Not content with their medical school, Jones and Bard went on to work for the establishment of a hospital and in March 1770, a petition was presented to the Lieutenant Governor, Cadwallader Colden. On his visit to London in that year John Jones raised money for the hospital, (no doubt with the help of John Fothergill) and it was Jones himself who drew the plans of an elegant eighteenth century building. The wards were to be thirty-six by twenty-four feet, with eight beds. Though it was burned while building in 1775, the hospital was opened in the following year. It makes a suitable memorial for John Jones, surgeon, patriot, teacher, who wrote in Hunterian style—'An operation alone is but a single point in the cure of disease' and 'the surgeon ought to have a mind calm and *intrepid* and yet humane and compassionate.'

By their names you may know this family of Welsh Americans, Wynne, Cadwalader and Jones. These men were not Welshmen, though descended from Wales, their families having left their ancient heritage for a new, more confident land. They were Americans, and American patriots.

I acknowledge gratefully the assistance given by Miss Jessie Dobson, late Curator of the Hunterian Museum, Royal College of Surgeons of England : Mr B. G. Owens, Keeper of Manuscripts and Records, National Library of Wales, Aberystwyth : and W. B. McDaniel 2nd, Curator of Historical Collections, Library of the College of Physicians of Philadelphia.

REFERENCES

Bell, W. J. (1965) *John Morgan Continental Doctor*. University of Pennsylvania, Philadelphia.

Blackwell, H. *Dictionary of Welsh Biography*. National Library of Wales. MSS. 9251-77.

Charles, S. T. (1965). John Jones, American Surgeon and Conservative Patriot. *Bull. Hist Med.*, 39, 435.

Felton, J. S. (1969). Thomas Cadwalader, M.D., Physician, Philadelphian and Philanthropist. *J. Occup. Med.*, 11. 374-380.

Garrison, F. H. (1929). *An Introduction to the History of Medicine*, 4th ed., p. 303. Saunders, Philadelphia.

Glenn, T. A. (1911). *Welsh Founders of Pennsylvania*, Vol. 1, pp. 20, 21 and 151. Fox, Jones & Co., Oxford.

Jones, J. (1776). *Plain Concise, Practical Remarks on the Treatment of Wounds and Fractures*. Bell, Philadelphia.

Holmes, O. W. (1883). *Medical Essays*, 1842-1882. Houghton Mifflin & Co., Boston.

Maxwell, J. P. (1930). Further Studies in Osteomalacia. *Proc. R. Soc. Med.*, 23, 639-652.

Mease, J. (1828). John Jones. In Thacher, J. (1828), Vol. 1, p. 324.

Middleton, W. S. (1941). Thomas Cadwalader and his Essay. *Ann. Med. Hist.* 3 s., 3, 101-113.

Peltier, L. F. (1966). John Jones : An Extraordinary American. *Surgery*, 59. 631-635.

Penrhyn Jones, G. (1960) Cadwalader and Bevan. *Lancet*, 1, 827.

Ruschenberger, W. S. W. (1887). *An Account of the Institution and Progress of the College of Physicians of Philadelphia during a Hundred Years, from January* 1787. Dornan, Philadelphia.

Salmon, D. (1924). The Quakers of Pembrokeshire. *Trans. hist. Soc. W. Wales*, 9.

Stookey, (1962). *A History of Colonial Medical Education in the Province of New York, with its subsequent development* (1767-1830). Charles C Thomas, Springfield, Illinois. passim.

Thacher, J. (1827). *A Military Journal during the American Revolutionary War. To which is added an appendix containing biographical sketches of several General Officers*, 2nd ed. Cottons and Barnard, Boston.

Thacher, J. (1828). *American Medical Biography*. 2 vols. Richardson and Lord, etc. Boston.

Viets, H. (1930). *A Brief History of Medicine in Massachusetts*. Houghton Mifflin & Co., Boston.

THE NEW MEDICAL CENTRE AND THE DEVELOPMENT OF MEDICAL EDUCATION IN WALES

A. Trevor Jones

At this British Congress on the History of Medicine which takes place in Wales, it is especially appropriate to give some account of the development of medical education in Wales. It is also a privilege to speak to the Congress within this new complex in Cardiff which we call the *Medical Teaching Centre,* the most recent achievement in the progress of School and Hospitals. This implies, (as it is meant to imply) that the Welsh National School of Medicine and the University Hospital are complementary parts of one institution.

It is perhaps one of the more interesting functions of historians (and this includes medical historians) to seek in the turn of events the reasons for the evolution of a particular institution, be it a nation, a society or even a medical school. In medical history we can find, if we look for them, reasons for its contrasting ways of training doctors—in London, in Scotland, on the Continent of Europe, in the United States of America ; but medicine has always tended to be a *vocational* education rather than seeking the objectives of the mediaeval universities (*universitas*) which attempted to teach the whole range of knowledge. Pre-occupation with the manifestations of disease which were gathered together in hospitals—whether they were called leper-houses, asylums or hospices—was the motivation for finding out more about the causes of diseases, and teaching others how to treat them.

So it was in Cardiff. Outside the East Gate of the town, on the road to Newport, the *Domus Leprosum* of St Mary Magdalen was established in the fourteenth century, a house providing beds for '24 leprous persons, poor and feeble folk' (Rees 1969). The Spital, as it was called, did not survive the Reformation and it was by chance that this same site was chosen by Daniel Jones of Beaupre for a new

Infirmary (Plate 1) which was founded in 1837, taking the place of an earlier public dispensary in Crockherbtown (now Queen Street). In laying the Foundation Stone (still preserved in the doorway of the present Royal Infirmary) Daniel Jones then said,

> Cardiff is a rising place and likely to become a Port of great trade and opulence. When the people of the hills are likewise considered and who may also partake of the benefits of this institution, this building must be looked upon as one of vast importance and advantage.

At that time Cardiff had a population of only seven thousand served by seven doctors, and came second after Merthyr Tydfil as the metropolis of south Wales and indeed Merthyr was better served medically than Cardiff. The Infirmary at that time had only twenty beds, with very primitive utilities, even without main drainage, until 1849. Piped water was brought in 1853, and gas in 1856.

From this time onwards Cardiff, with better communications, first by canal and later by railway, had expanded to a considerable town of 90,000 and by 1880 the Infirmary, in spite of additions, could not keep pace with demands ; it was grossly overcrowded and was subject to the then inevitable outbreaks of communicable diseases (Plate 2). The only solution was to move to new and larger buildings. These were completed by 1883 on an open site on Longcross Common (Plate 3) ; these later became known as the Cardiff Royal Infirmary and were destined to become eventually the first home of the clinical departments of the medical school. But the old Infirmary had made its contribution to medicine and medical education, for here in 1870 was founded the Cardiff Medical Society—one of the oldest in the country—which provided a forum for lively discussions on medical subjects. The active members of this society continually pressed for a medical school in Cardiff, and this coincided with the moves which were taking place in education generally in Wales, which included the clamant desire for a Welsh university.

It may possibly surprise many that the university of Wales is one of the oldest, and comes fifth after Oxford and Cambridge, Durham and London. I except of course, those institutions in Scotland, whose origins were largely municipal, and began more as a means of comprehensive education for the active inquirers after knowledge in those ancient burghs. But in Wales, the impetus for a university came from

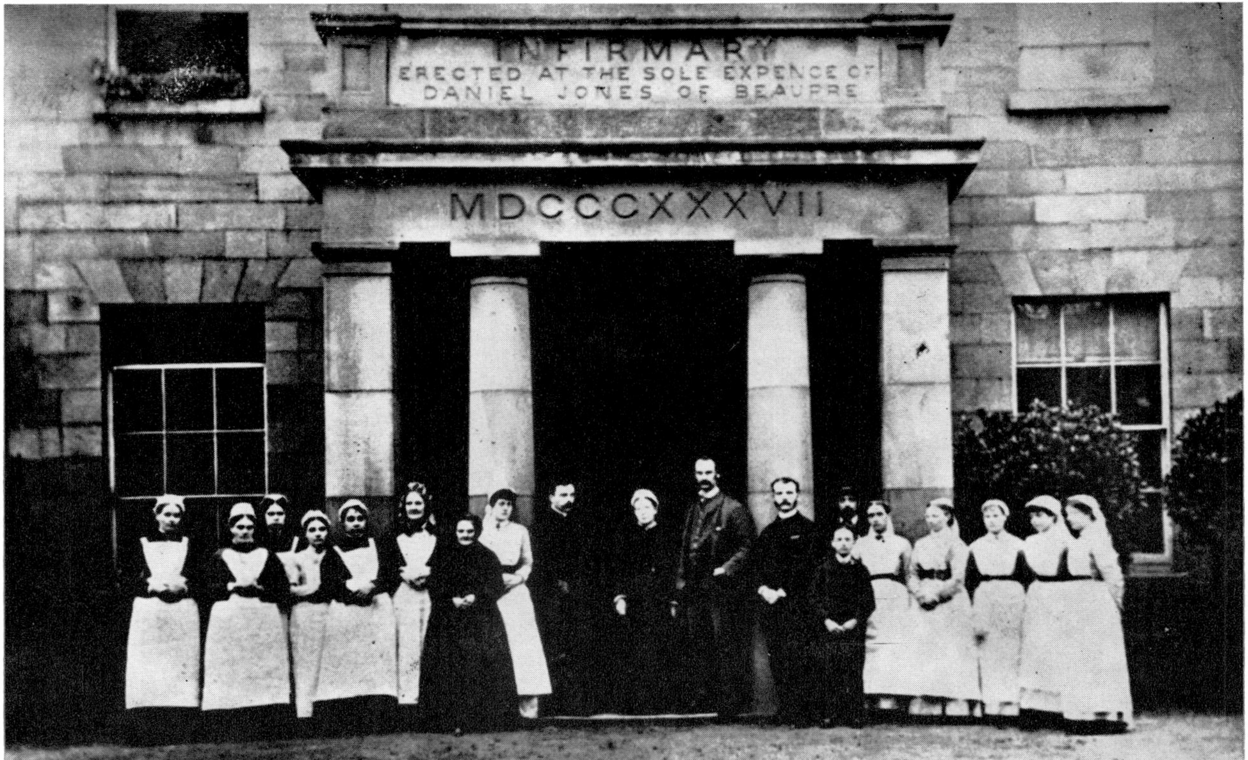
INFIRMARY
ERECTED AT THE SOLE EXPENCE OF
DANIEL JONES OF BEAUPRE
MDCCCXXXVII

Plate 1
The "Old" Infirmary built in 1837

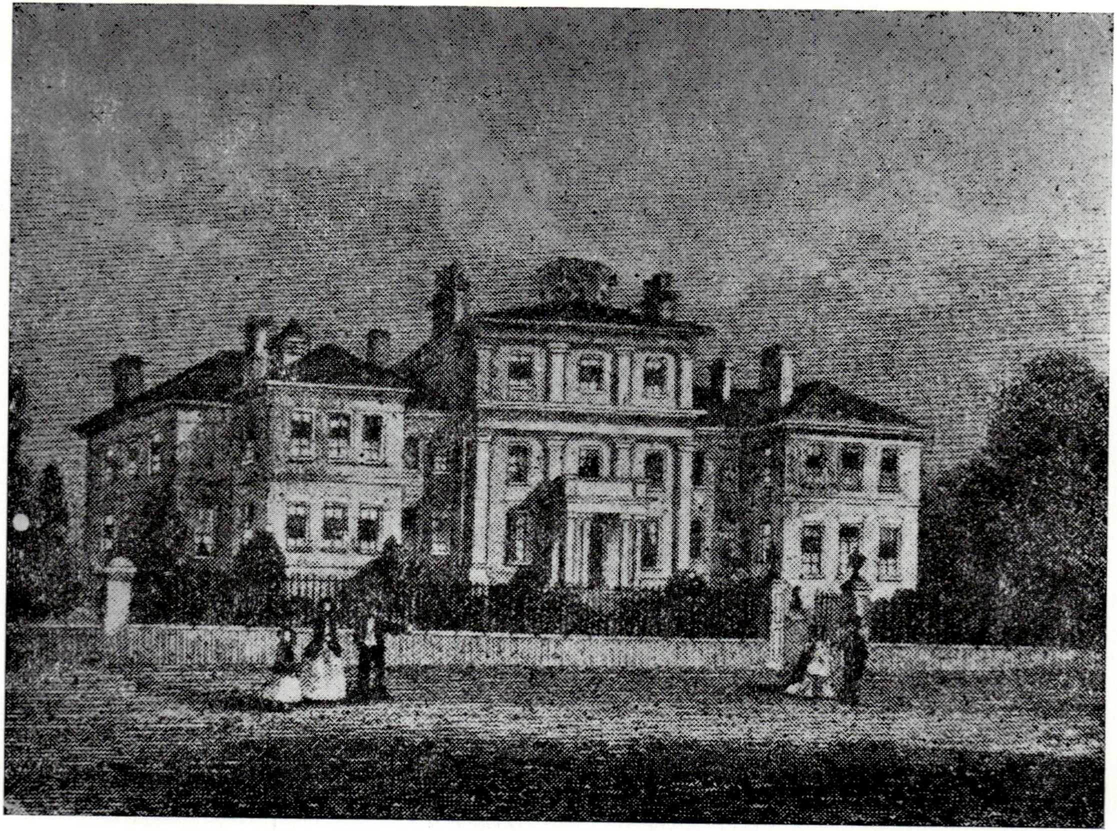

Plate 2
Glamorganshire and Monmouthshire Infirmary 1865

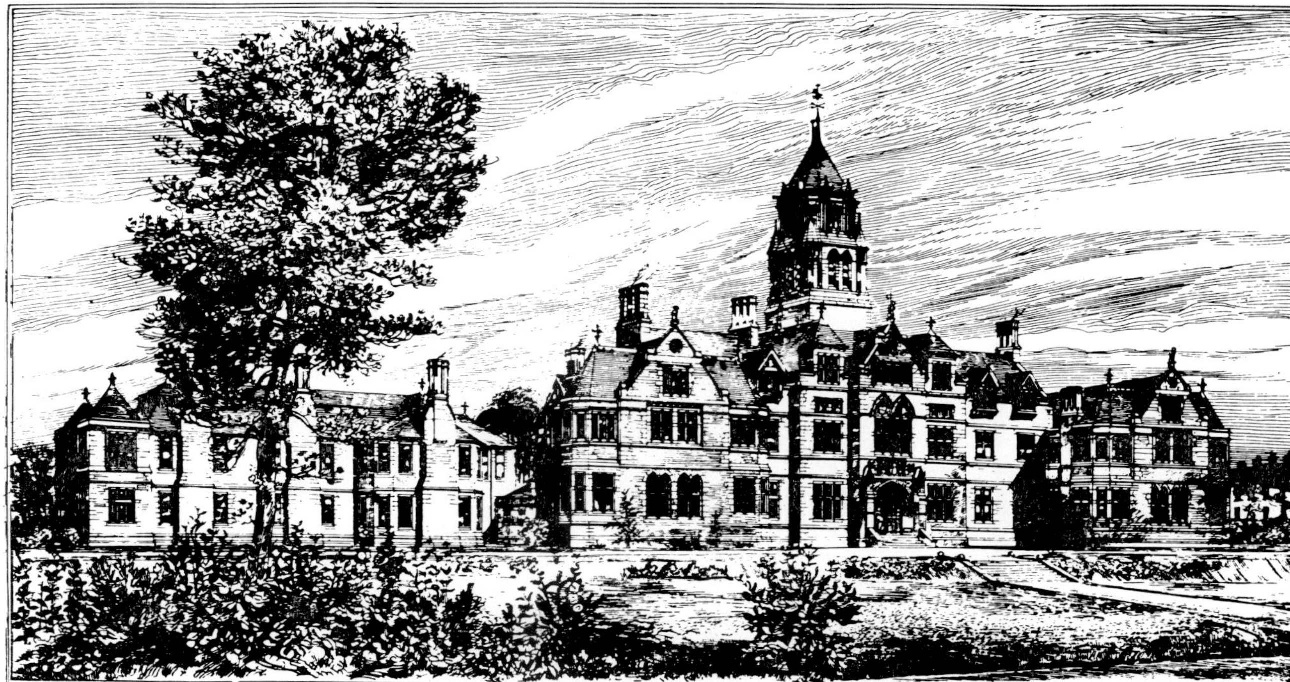

Plate 3
Cardiff Infirmary 1883

those who envisaged a national academy which the intelligent of all classes could attend without crossing the border. Included in these proposals was a school of medicine, but the middle of the last century was hardly the period when help was likely to come from public sources. Support had to be solicited from private benefactors and contributions from working people. Moreover the very geography of Wales presented formidable problems (as it still does !) but in spite of many frustrations, difficulties and disappointments, teaching colleges were established first in Aberystwyth in 1872, in Bangor, north Wales in 1880, and in Cardiff in 1883. An indication of the financial stress is shown by the fact that in each of these places, the colleges had to make do with a 'second-hand' building : in Aberystwyth a bankrupt holiday hotel was used, and in Bangor the college made its first home in an old hostelry on the Holyhead Road. In Cardiff, our two stories come together, for the old Daniel Jones Infirmary, vacated for the move to the new site already mentioned, became in 1883—with the goodwill of all concerned—the seat of the University College of South Wales and Monmouthshire. Indeed this old building with alterations and additions (' rabbit hutches ' as they were called by Tom Ellis), remained the only university establishment in south Wales for many years, for it was not until 1909 that the Cardiff College was able to open its fine new buildings on a site of five acres in Cathays Park forming part of the Civic Centre, which is so well known. But the 'Old College,' as it was affectionately known, continued in Newport Road, and among the additions were departments of anatomy and physiology, so that a faculty of medicine was established there in 1893, and by what seems now a significant coincidence hospital buildings became available for the teaching of medical subjects. A complete medical school using the nearby Royal Infirmary had always been the aim, but not until many years later (actually in 1921) was this achieved. During these 30 years Cardiff medical students had to proceed to London to complete their clinical studies, not without benefit (it may be claimed !) to the staffs and achievements of the university of London and its medical schools.

It was not surprising that the early years were periods of struggle ; the colleges were isolated from each other, finding even maintenance funds difficult to obtain, let alone capital for developments, and (except for Cardiff) were not sited in prosperous manufacturing cities as in England where the communities were proud to develop their own universities as independent institutions. Furthermore, the idea (one might almost call it an ideal) of a federal organisation appealed to the people of Wales where the ambition of a national culture was a patriotic aim. This inevitably led to the establishment of the University of Wales, with three constituent colleges, by royal charter in 1893, thereby securing its seniority over the many provincial universities in England, where, more particularly in recent years, there has been a rush (one may even call it a rash) of new establishments.

This is not to say that the Welsh university was free from stresses and strains—among the causes were not only its federal constitution, but also the demand for a complete medical school. In the midst of the First World War in 1916 a royal commission (Evans 1953) was set up under the chairmanship of Lord Haldane to consider the work of the university and the relations of the colleges. Included amongst its members were Sir William Osler, then Regius Professor of Medicine at Oxford, Sir William Bragg, Professor of Physics at University College, London, and other distinguished Welsh and English academics. The commission reported in 1918, making many recommendations and more relevant to this history, it proposed there should be a medical school at Cardiff to be counted among the constituent institutions of the university of Wales, directly responsible to its court. Also amongst its more interesting ideas (at least as far as medicine is concerned) was the adoption of the 'professorial unit' system, then a new concept in England, although later to be adopted by University College Hospital, London and now followed by all the medical schools in the country.

It was not to be expected that Cardiff College could welcome this amputation of its medical faculty with any enthusiasm, for after all, it had supported the pre-clinical departments for many years often at the expense of other departments ; so that when it was possible in 1921 to make a start on clinical education, the school remained as a part of the college. New professorial chairs and departments were established in addition to the existing departments of anatomy physiology, bacteriology, pathology and pharmacology. Notable among these chairs were those made possible by local benefactors : the Mansel-Talbot Chair in Hygiene and Public Health in 1919, and the David Davies Chair of Tuberculosis in 1921. But another complication was the insertion of the professorial units into the already congested Royal Infirmary, which at that time was the only general hospital in Cardiff. The medical unit was however, provided with a new building integrated in the infirmary by the benevolence of the Rockefeller Foundation, but the relations between the hospital and the college brought about a crisis in 1927, so that clinical education had to cease.

The stranded clinical students were rescued by the generosity of University College Hospital, London, a gesture which should never be forgotten. (Incidentally it should be mentioned that during the Second World War of 1939-45, this debt was gladly repaid by the Cardiff School by accepting evacuated students from U.C.H., together with their distinguished teachers, among whom were Thomas Lewis and Max Rosenheim).

The crisis of the twenties was eventually solved by the vigorous action of the university court, and in 1931 the Welsh National School of Medicine was established by charter, with its own council and senate, and with its own administrative head, the provost, co-equal in most respects, with the principals of the other colleges, which now included the new College of Swansea. The Cardiff College, however, retained its pre-clinical departments (Trow and Brown 1933), although academic and administrative links between the college and the school were preserved and were incorporated in their respective charters.

The school was now able to progress with its 'Recognised Clinical Institutions' which now included not only the Cardiff Royal Infirmary but also the newly built municipal hospital at Llandough, Whitchurch Mental Hospital and the institutions of the Welsh National Memorial Association for Tuberculosis. By a series of reciprocal arrangements with this variety of authorities, the staffs of these hospitals were recognised as clinical teachers, and the medical school staffs were given facilities for teaching in them.

At this time—even during a war—however, general consideration was being given to the way in which medical schools and teaching hospitals should be mobilised and organised for mutual benefit, and an inter-departmental committee (Goodenough 1944) produced valuable guide lines for the future. Moreover the war time government had already committed the country to a Health Service for the Nation in October 1941. A series of hospital surveys carried out for the Minister of Health towards the end of the war included a Report for South Wales (Jones, Nixon and Picken 1945) which recognised the need for a completely new teaching hospital in Cardiff on a new site ; for, as the surveyors said

> No plan will be of any avail unless there is a reasonable certainty that the requisite numbers of highly trained medical, nursing and other personnel can be obtained.

All this time, before, during and after the war, teaching and medical school departments in Cardiff had to be improvised within the hospitals, and there is no doubt that these arrangements influenced the authorities and staffs towards the advantages of close integration of teaching and research on the one hand with clinical care on the other. It was this policy which was followed by the several authorities who set about the work of completing a new teaching hospital and school in Cardiff. These authorities were the University, the School and College and the newly constituted Hospital Boards (under the N.H.S. Act 1946) who set up Joint Working Parties. Negotiations with Cardiff Corporation resulted in the availability of a convenient site of 53 acres at Heath Park, on which a medical school, with a greatly increased entry, a dental school, a hospital of 800 beds together with schools for the ancillary professions could all be accommodated.

Schedules of accommodation were prepared, which were to form the basis of an architectural competition ; for this was to be a new type of venture in which two governmental agencies (viz the University Grants Committee and the Ministry of Health) were concerned, and consequently the relationships, harmonious though they were, had to be meticulously regulated. It was not until 1962 that we were allowed to go ahead with the site contract. The first stage, the Dental School and Hospital was completed by 1965, and the final phases by 1971 (Plate 4), which, considering the size of the project (about 1,200,000 sq. ft.) can be considered as satisfactory.

This is not the place to go into the details of the plans and design, for they are described in a publication by the University of Wales Press (Surtees and Jones 1971) but the main feature is the closest integration of academic facilities with the clinical services, combined with easy communications and the possibility for future alterations. The advantages of concentration in one large institution (Plate 5) are sometimes apt to be forgotten, of course, and the inevitable changes, improvements, and additions will be matched, it is hoped, by changes in the attitudes of those who will be concerned with its function.

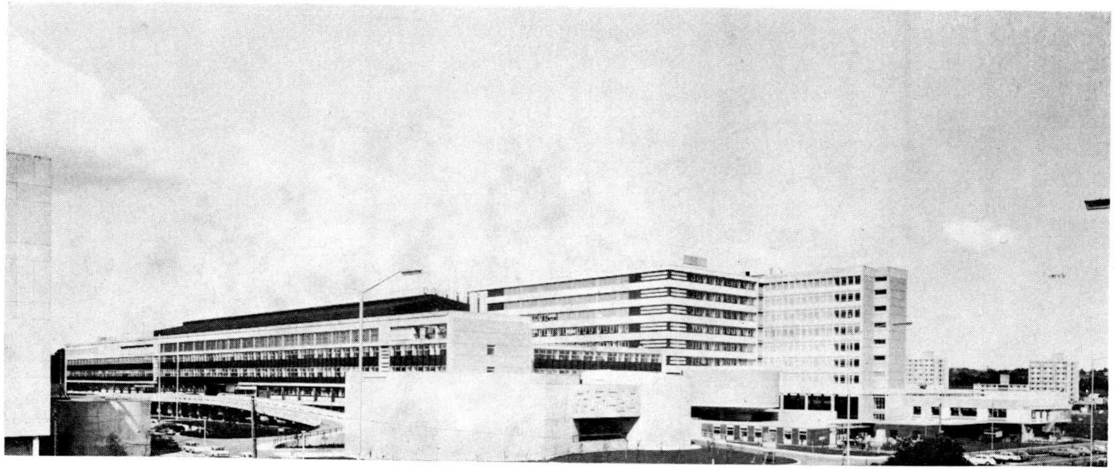

Plate 4
The Welsh National School of Medicine and the University Hospital of Wales

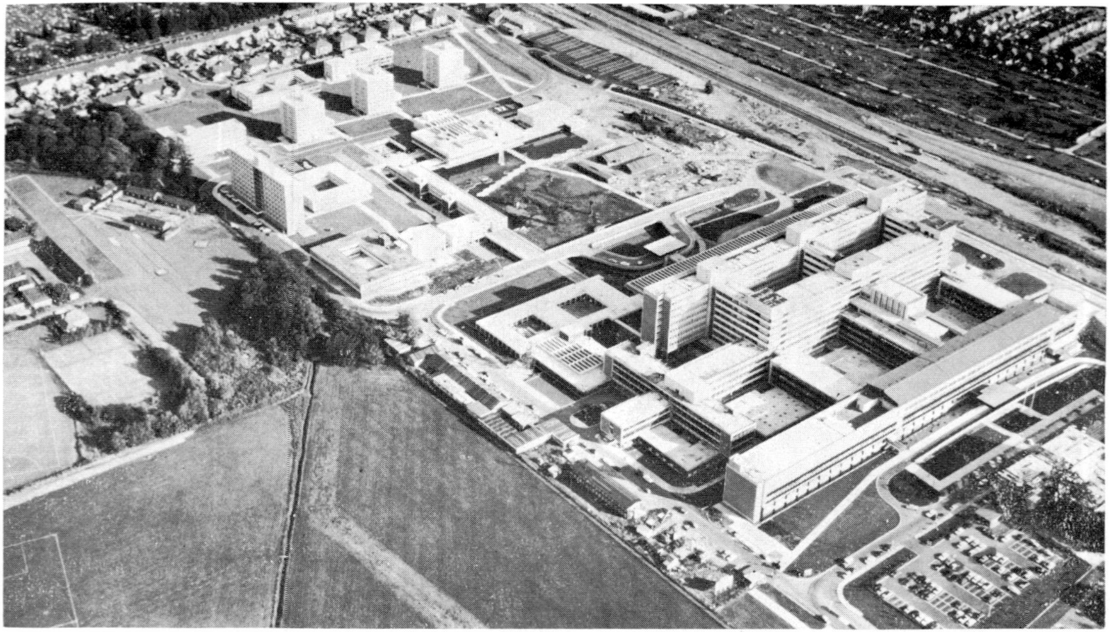

Plate 5
Aerial view of the Medical Teaching Centre

Among the more important features is the accommodation for the teaching and training of the many ancillary workers in the Health Services, already recognised as of increasing importance ; perhaps it is too early to hope that the university will take them under its wing, but in the future, enlightened academic institutions will realise that vocational training is as respectable now as it was in the Middle Ages. It is also important to realise that hospital diagnosis and treatment should be complementary to health activities in the community. This had been recognised by the School in establishing a general practice health centre in a nearby new estate in Cardiff where medical and dental students can be introduced to the needs of general practice in its widest sense, and where the staff can carry out postgraduate teaching, and study at first hand the health and social problems of the community.

History is traditionally concerned with the past, but its lessons should, and sometimes do, hold clues to the future. The evolvement of medical education shows that changes cannot be foreseen, but those concerned should keep alert for any alterations in the real needs, as opposed to popular demands, of society generally.

REFERENCES

Evans, D. E. (1953). *The University of Wales : a Historical Sketch,* Chap. 3. University of Wales Press, Cardiff.

Ibid. Chap. 9.

Goodenough, W., *et al.* (1944). *Report of the Inter-Departmental Committee on Medical Schools.* H.M.S.O., London.

Jones, A. T., Nixon, J. A., and Picken, R.M.F. (1945). *Hospital Survey : The Hospital Services of South Wales and Monmouthshire.* H.M.S.O., London.

Rees, W. (1969) *Cardiff : a History of the City,* 2nd ed. p. 22. Cardiff City Corporation, Cardiff.

Surtees, J. and Jones, A. T., (1971). *The Medical Teaching Centre Cardiff,* University of Wales Press, Cardiff.

Trow, A. H., and Brown D. J. A. (1933). *A Short History of the College,* pp. 59-64. Western Mail and Echo, Cardiff.

THE KING EDWARD VII WELSH NATIONAL MEMORIAL ASSOCIATION
1912—1948

GLYNNE R. JONES

'*If curable, why not cured?*'—Edward VII referring to tuberculosis.

INTRODUCTION

Tuberculosis remained the commonest single cause of death in Wales at the beginning of this century,[1] despite a gradual decline in mortality since the mid nineteenth century.[2] Respecting neither creed nor social class tuberculosis was 'the most widespread of all diseases and the most devastating in its ravages upon the manpower of the United Kingdom'.[3] However, apart from a few isolated instances, no facilities were available for its comprehensive treatment in Wales. Notable exceptions were the Manchester Board of Guardians Sanatorium at Abergele, Denbs., (1906),[4] a block erected at Allt-yr-Yn Hospital, Newport (1906) by the Corporation [5] and the West Wales Sanatorium at Alltymynydd, Llanybyther, Carms., (1908)[6] built by voluntary effort.

Remembering the numerous memorial clocks and fountains erected after the death of Queen Victoria, David Davies, M.P. of Llandinam conceived the idea of a more objective Welsh memorial to the late King Edward VII.[7] At a national conference of public bodies held at Shrewsbury on 30th September 1910 it was decided that the Memorial should be a national campaign to eradicate tuberculosis from Wales and Monmouthshire.[8] Subsequently, at public meetings convened by the Lords Lieutenant in each Welsh county, public interest in the tuberculosis problem was stimulated[8] and a starting capital of over £200,000 was raised.[9]

The National Insurance Act 1911 was amended to enable Welsh local authorities to delegate their obligation to provide an anti-tuberculosis service to the Memorial, and the local authorities hemselves provided finance from the rates.[8, 10] The royal charter granted on 17th May 1912 marked the beginning of the King Edward VII Welsh National Memorial Association for the prevention, treatment and abolition of tuberculosis (W.N.M.A.).[11] There was wide representation on its board of governors, including the Treasury, the Local Government Board, the Welsh Insurance Commissioners, the Medical Officers of Health, the County and County Borough Councils, corporate bodies, Trade Unions and others.[12]

THE EARLY YEARS (1912—1918)

The W.N.M.A. provided a unified comprehensive anti-tuberculosis service with equal facilities throughout Wales, that was available free to workers and non-workers.[11] An education programme on the principles of prevention preceded the treatment of patients ; indeed the public lecturers and travelling exhibitions[13] became commonplace in the Principality during the next thirty-six years. This campaign dispelled the popular belief that tuberculosis was a hereditary disease incapable of influence by man.

Controlled from the head office in Cardiff, with a central bacteriological laboratory, Wales was divided into thirteen districts, each with a central dispensary and outlying visiting stations, in the charge of an independent experienced tuberculosis physician assisted by a tuberculosis nurse. Tuberculosis hospital beds owned or rented by the W.N.M.A. were available in each district, while the sanatoria with their more specialized role served a wider area.[14] Beds at several hospitals in England were also used by the Association.[15]

Dr Marcus Paterson, the first medical director was formerly head of Frimley Sanatorium and had an international reputation for his methods of treating tuberculosis.[16] Clinical work began in July 1912 ; initially, only those with advanced disease were referred, reflecting the reluctance of the general practitioners or the sufferers to use the new facilities.[17] The problem was a formidable one ; tuberculosis was found in 70 % of adults and 43 % of children examined,[18] while in contacts 30 % of adults and 21 % of children also had the disease.[19] The prevalence of infection is further exemplified by the finding that of 348 sputum specimens obtained from public footpaths in Swansea in 1914, tubercle bacilli were present in 57 %.[20]

The enthusiasm of the W.N.M.A. staff ensured real progress from the outset by overcoming public prejudice to those suffering from tuberculosis, controlling the spread of infection, and rehabilitating the patients both mentally and physically.[21] However, the Great War brought with it familiar problems—rising costs,[22] insufficient hospital beds[23] and staff shortages (a third of the medical staff served with the Armed Forces)[24, 25] in the face of an increasing workload. Despite all of this the W.N.M.A. continued to expand and provide an improved service.[26]

THE PEMBROKESHIRE SAGA

There were local administrative difficulties too. In 1912 all local authorities had agreed to join the W.N.M.A. scheme, though Carmarthenshire and Breconshire, pending clarification of the financial arrangements, did not participate fully until 1913 and 1917 respectively.[27, 28] Pembrokeshire alone remained aloof demanding the right for their medical officer of health to exercise control over the tuberculosis physician, dispensaries and tuberculosis hospitals within the county.[29] The W.N.M.A. would not accept any compromise in providing a unified comprehensive service ;[30] facilities continued to be provided in Pembrokeshire under considerable difficulties and for financial reasons were restricted to those persons insured under the National Insurance Act, 1911. The alternative scheme submitted by Pembrokeshire for the treatment of tuberculosis within the county was not accepted by the Welsh Insurance Commissioners,[31] while the crude death rate for the disease there was 1570 per million population, greater than the national average. It was not until 1920 that Pembrokeshire, having no practical alternative, finally rejoined the W.N.M.A. and paid arrears.[32]

BETWEEN THE WARS (1919—1938)

After the First World War the service was expanded and facilities extended. (Table) New hospitals were built or bought in many parts of Wales,[33] the most notable being the North Wales Sanatorium at Llangwyfan, Denbs (226 beds) and the South Wales Sanatorium at Talgarth, Brecs (304 beds—the largest in the United Kingdom), both of which were officially opened by King George V and Queen Mary in July 1920.[34] Over thirty distinguished consulting staff gave their services part-time to the W.N.M.A., including Sir Robert Philip, Sir Thomas Lewis, Sir Robert Jones, Sir John Lynn-Thomas, Sir

TABLE

REPRESENTATIVE W.N.M.A. STATISTICS DURING THE PERIOD 1912 TO 1948[1]

	1912	1915	1920	1925	1930	1935	1940	1945	1948
Total attendances at clinics	3240[2]	9155	12616	12970	44484	47016	60921	107856	129687
Number of new patients examined					13164	13177	17623	33392	38015
Crude death rate per million	1291	1464	1226	1106	977	925	796	718	630
Number of medical staff (whole time)	20	25[3]	28	40	39	46	42[4]	42	46
Hospital beds owned by W.N.M.A.	200[5]	603	1128	1400	1410	1516	1827	2111	2107
Hospital beds rented by W.N.M.A.	179[5]	983	78	28	100	149	182	511	537
Beds vacant through staff shortage								425	356
Net annual cost of W.N.M.A. scheme	£21196[2]	£86306	£132997	£184784	£198465	£238627	£355159	£467691	£608748[6]

1 Taken from the W.N.M.A. Annual Reports
2 Period July 1912 to March 1913
3 Nine of these were serving with the Armed Forces
4 Three of these were serving with the Armed forces
5 Approximate numbers
6 Cost for period March 1947 to March 1948

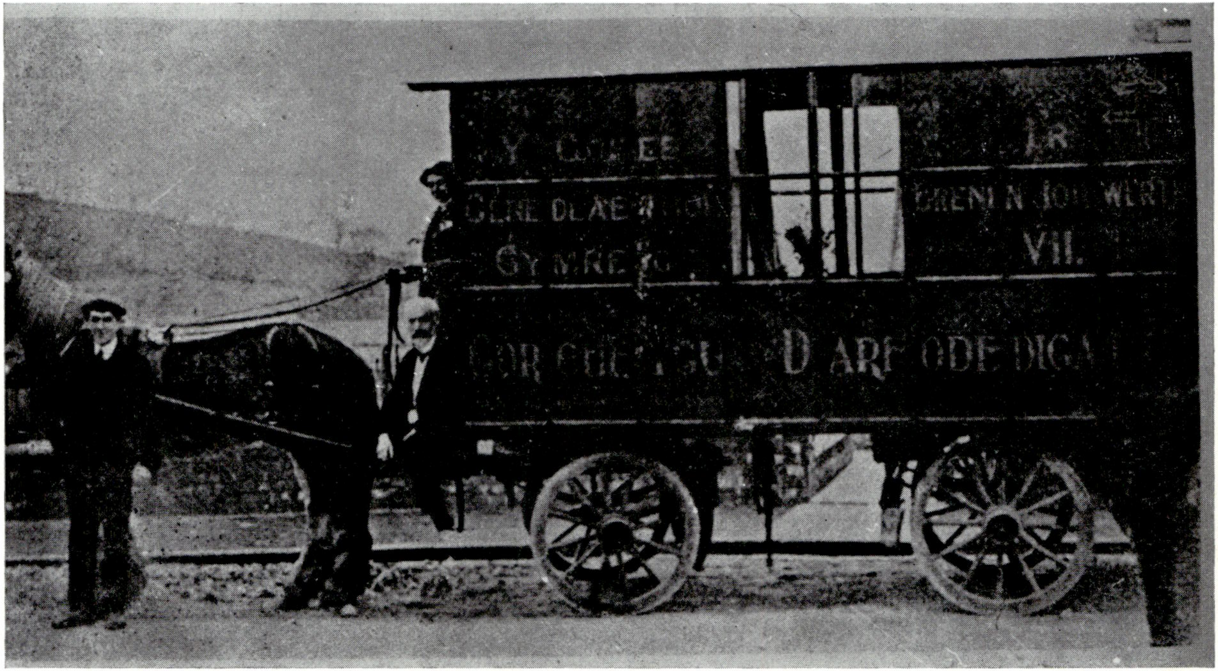

Plate 6

The horse-drawn caravan and team which toured Wales in the early days advertising the work of the W.N.M.A., Dr R. Owen Morris, Superintendent of the educational campaign seated. (W.N.M.A. Annual Report 1910–1913).

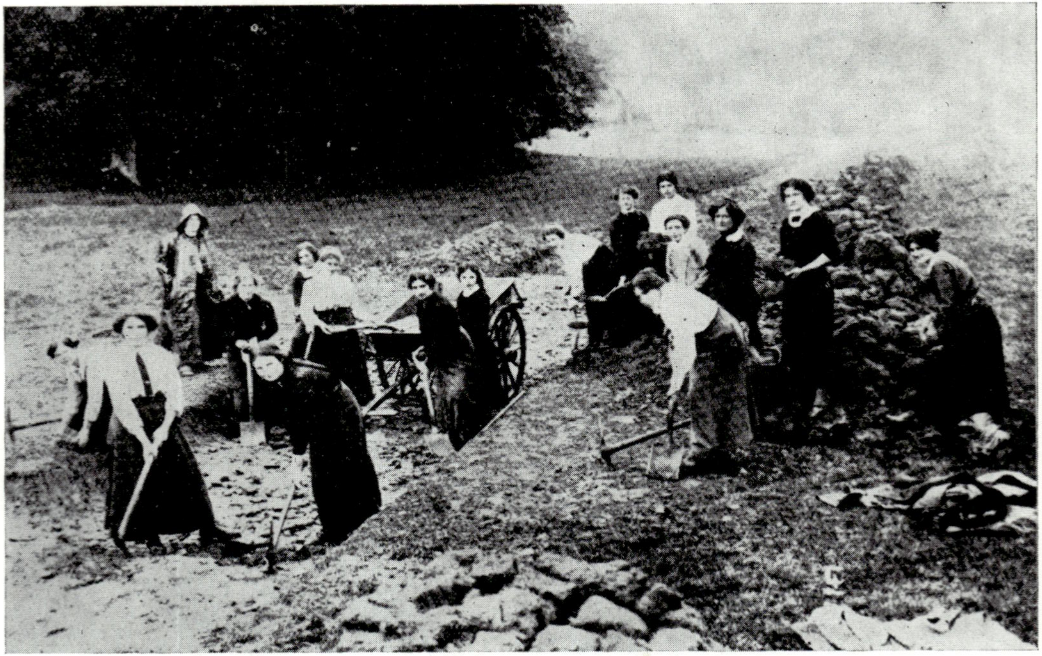

Plate 7

Graduated labour. Women patients working at the South Wales Sanatorium, Talgarth, constructing a road to the new Sanatorium buildings. (W.N.M.A. Annual Report 1914).

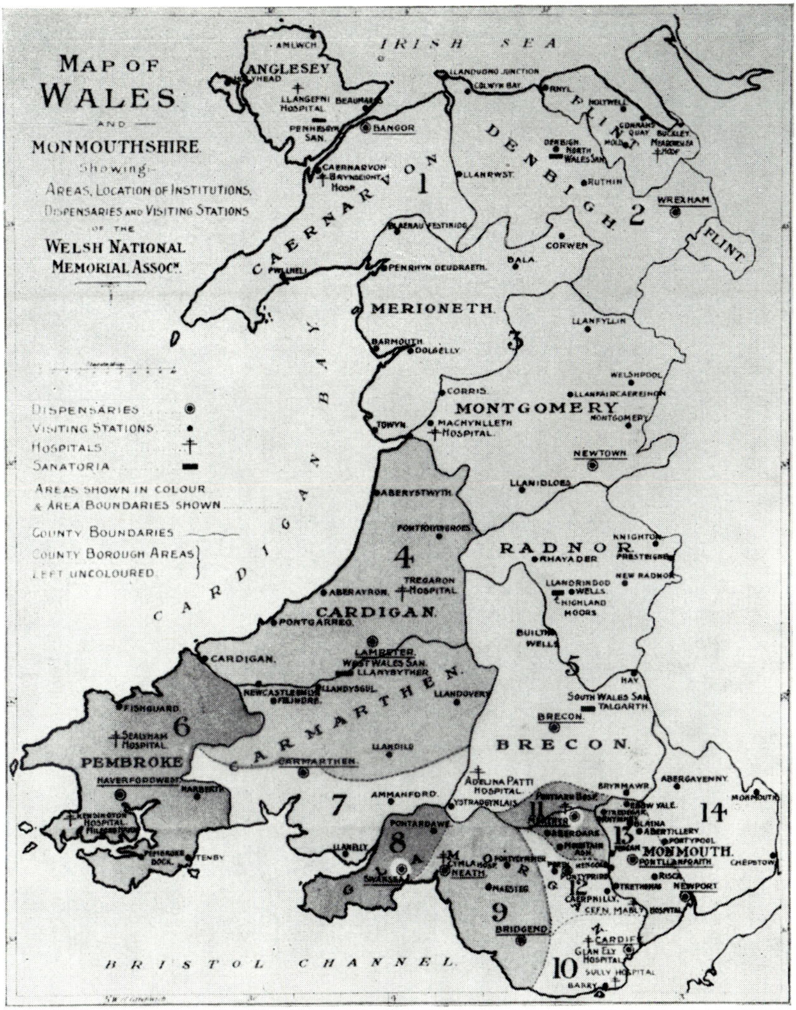

Plate 8
Map showing Areas, locations of Institutions, Dispensaries and Visiting Stations of the W.N.M.A.
(W.N.M.A. Annual Report 1936).

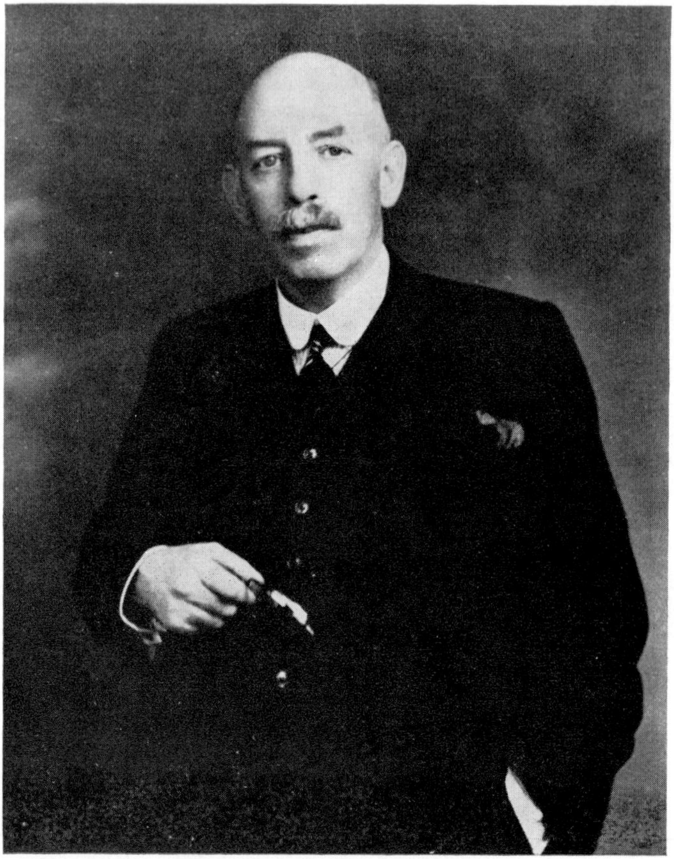

Plate 9
David Davies of Llandinam.
President of the W.N.M.A. from 1912 to 1944.
(Courtesy of Dr H. M. Foreman, Sully Hospital).

Henry Gauvain, Mr Morriston Davies and the clinical professors of the Welsh National School of Medicine.[35]

New methods of diagnosis and treatment were introduced and evaluated by the W.N.M.A. ;[36] radiography,[37, 38] ultraviolet light for skin tuberculosis and sinuses,[39–41] surgical treatment of bone and joint and genito-urinary tuberculosis,[42] and various forms of collapse therapy for pulmonary tuberculosis [43,44]—with dramatic results. The W.N.M.A. provided a unique opportunity for co-ordinated multicentre research ; the epidemiology of tuberculosis in different Welsh communities,[45–51] the trial in conjunction with the Medical Research Council of various drugs and vaccines thought to have anti-tuberculous activity,[52–54] an evaluation of the tuberculin reactions[55, 56] and the investigation of the pathology and radiology of coal-workers' pneumoconiosis[57, 58] were amongst the projects. The appendix lists some of the research papers written by the W.N.M.A. staff.

The educational campaign was directed primarily at school children (as many as 87,000 children being addressed annually[59]) and other selected groups such as teachers and university students. The W.N.M.A. pressed for tuberculosis-free milk[60] and meat, and were instrumental in obtaining power, through the Public Health Act, 1925, for the compulsory institutional treatment of patients with open pulmonary tuberculosis considered to be a danger to the community.[61]

In 1920 the David Davies Chair of Tuberculosis at the Welsh National School of Medicine was endowed by David Davies and his sisters in memory of their grandfather ;[62] the postgraduate course leading to the Tuberculosis Diseases Diploma (T.D.D.) of the University of Wales was established three years later.[63] The first Professor, Col. S. Lyle Cummins (formerly professor of pathology at the Royal Army Medical College) was both a clinical teacher in the Welsh National School of Medicine, and director of research to the W.N.M.A.,[64] thus closely linking the medical school with the Association.

By 1932 the W.N.M.A. with twenty years' experience behind it was running smoothly and coping with an ever increasing volume of work (Table).[65] The annual running costs were £200,000,[66] less than elsewhere in the United Kingdom for a comparable area and population ; a sanatorium bed cost a mere £2 per week to maintain.[67] There were now seventeen institutions providing a total of 1487 beds, a further 110 beds being rented,[68] fourteen dispensary areas and over one hundred visiting stations ;[69] the whole-time staff including all doctors, nurses teachers, domestics and administrators totalled 881.[70] Over 194,000 people had been examined since 1912, of whom 74,500 were suffering from tuberculosis,[70] and though the death rate continued to fall, the disease still accounted for some 17% of all deaths in Wales.[71]

The medical emphasis in hospital was being extended from sanatorium treatment for limited disease, to include active surgical intervention in advanced disease. This required more hospital beds with surgical facilities, and this necessary expansion was increasingly hampered by rising costs (Table). Sully Hospital (300 beds), the last to be built by the W.M.N.A., was opened by the Duke of Kent in 1936[72] for the surgical treatment of tuberculosis ; here visiting consultant surgeons like Sir Clement Price Thomas operated at weekends in the early days, while the resident staff were being trained in the new techniques.

Though continual reorganisation and reassessment resulted in an increased efficiency and effectiveness, the W.N.M.A. was not without criticism. The death rate from tuberculosis in Wales still exceeded that in England, and there were objections also to the W.N.M.A. policies for expenditure.[73] This culminated in the inquiry by the Ministry of Health into the anti-tuberculosis service in Wales and Monmouthshire (1938),[10] which found that the W.M.N.A. facilities for the diagnosis and treatment of tuberculosis were satisfactory though there was some shortage of beds ; the main criticism was of the failure of the Local Authorities to implement fully preventive measures in conjunction with the W.N.M.A.[74] This comprehensive report had far reaching social and environmental implications, and resulted in closer co-operation between the W.N.M.A. and the various local authorities. As there were still no effective antituberculous drugs available, prevention of the disease through education was imperative ; the W.N.M.A. bilingual educational film 'The Crusade', released in 1935, was probably the first 'talkie' to have a Welsh commentary.[75]

THE LATTER YEARS (1939—1948)

The outbreak of the Second World War accentuated the difficulties of the W.N.M.A., the embargo on all capital expenditure prohibiting further expansion of the service.[76] Emergency medical service beds at their own institutions, and those at Abergavenny, Chepstow and Morriston (Swansea) were made available to the Association when not in use,[77] to combat a work-load that increased more rapidly than ever before,[78], [79] though the acute staff shortage during and after the war years forced the closure of beds at some of the W.N.M.A. hospitals (Table).[77], [80]

However, in the midst of adversity the W.N.M.A. launched the first mobile Miniature Mass Radiography (M.M.R.) unit in the United Kingdom (February, 1944),[81] in an attempt to make the diagnosis of tuberculosis at an earlier stage in the disease. The unit was capable of X-raying over one hundred persons per hour,[81] and within two years of its inception, over 100,000 people had been X-rayed ; of these some 0.5 % had tuberculosis and a further 2 % had some other chest condition.[82]

In 1944 too, David Davies of Llandinam died at the age of sixty-four.[83] Created first Baron Davies of Llandinam in 1932,[84] he was a man with many public interests at an international level ; his enthusiasm and generosity had enusred that the W.N.M.A. was a functional national memorial to King Edward VII. He built the Welsh National Temple of Peace and Health at Cardiff, completed in 1938 at a cost of £70,000,[85] which he later gave to the W.N.M.A. as their new headquarters.[86] It is ironic that the first X-ray taken by the M.M.R. unit when the campaign was launched in 1944 revealed Lord Davies to be suffering from an incurable condition from which he died shortly afterwards. He was succeeded as president of the W.N.M.A, by his son, Major Lord Davies, the second baron who was killed in action three months later ; the presidency passed finally to Miss Gwendoline Davies, C.H., sister of the first baron.[87]

The W.N.M.A. began the post war period working to full capacity and continued to provide a comprehensive service in addition to coping with the extra burdens placed on staff and resources by the M.M.R. unit (Table). With over three thousand patients waiting for beds, the shortage had reached desperate proportions ;[88] negotiations for a hospital site at Singleton Park, Swansea were completed,[89] and another site at Carmarthen was considered.[90]

However, great changes in the field of tuberculosis were imminent The tuberculosis physician had gradually become a chest physician and now dealt with industrial and other pulmonary disorders besides tuberculosis, particularly since the inception of the M.M.R. unit. In 1947 streptomycin was on trial by the Medical Research Council for the treatment of tuberculous meningitis, miliary disease and acute bilateral pulmonary tuberculosis,[91] followed early in 1948 by the trial of streptomycin and para-amino salicylic acid (P.A.S.) at Sully Hospital;[92] here for the first time was a treatment capable of curing more than 60% of patients suffering from tuberculosis.

Unfortunately perhaps, these were the twilight years, for the National Health Service Act 1946 sealed the fate of the W.N.M.A. The request of the Association to be left intact as a single regional unit with responsibility for tuberculosis within the new National Health Service was not granted.[93, 94] On 5th July, 1948 all institutions and staff of the W.N.M.A. were transferred to the Minister of Health and the new Welsh Regional Hospital Board,[95] who set up their offices in the W.N.M.A. headquarters at the Temple of Peace and Health, Cardiff.

Members of the former staff remember their years of service in the W.N.M.A. with pride. The quarterly medical staff meetings which began in 1914,[24] where the tuberculosis physicians discussed their problems and informed colleagues of research in progress, continued after 1948 and became embodied in the Thoracic Society of Wales with whom the tradition of the W.N.M.A. now rests.

IN RETROSPECT

The W.N.M.A. provided a hospital and domiciliary specialist service with complete responsibility for dealing with tuberculosis that was outstanding in its scope and quality. It is doubtful whether this measure of success would have been achieved had a smaller area been chosen for its operations. The Association proved that efficient management in the field of medicine was practicable for the whole of Wales and Monmouthshire treated as a single unit,[96] and provided an unique administrative model for the new National Health Service with specialist staff experienced in chest diseases and tuberculosis and a network of adequately equipped hospitals and clinics. Without precedent for guidance, the W.N.M.A. had overcome many unforseen obstacles and problems during its thirty-six years of existence, and appreciated the importance of enthusiasm, concentrated effort devotion to duty, co-ordination and co-operation at all levels both within and without the Association; indeed their own principal shortcoming had been the failure of a system whereby responsibility for the diagnosis and treatment of tuberculosis rested with one authority and the responsibility for preventive measures with another.[96]

There were few families in Wales without reason for gratitude to the W.N.M.A., which had grown to be the foremost anti-tuberculosis organisation in the British Empire, if not in the world—a fitting memorial to a king, which has ensured the W.N.M.A. of a place of honour in Welsh history.

ACKNOWLEDGEMENT

I am indebted to the former Tuberculosis Physician for Carmarthenshire, Dr John T. Jones (my father) for inspiration, and to Mrs S. M. Clark for typing the manuscript.

REFERENCES

(Note: *W.N.M.A. Ann. Rep.*—Annual Report of the King Edward VII Welsh National Memorial Association).

1 *W.N.M.A. Ann. Rep.* (1920), 8, 23.
2 McKeown, T. and Lowe, C. R. (1966) *An Introduction to Social Medicine*. Blackwell, Oxford, p. 9.
3 *W.N.M.A. Ann. Rep.* (1917), 5, 13. This quotes the Report by a Committee of Members of Parliament on the administration of Public Health, headed by Waldorf Astor, M.P., entitled 'The Health of the People'.
4 Jones, G. P. (1962) *Newyn a Haint yng Nghymru*. Llyfrfa'r Methodistiaid Calfinaidd, Caernarvon, p. 120.
5 *W.N.M.A. Ann. Rep.* (1943), 31. President's address.
6 James, D. H. (1908) *A Guide to Llanybyther and a Short History of the Foundation of Alltymynydd Sanatorium*. D. Jones, Pencader, p. 28.
7 Ross, H. A. (1957) "Long Ago". Unpublished MS in author's collection.
8 *W.N.M.A. Ann. Rep.* (1910–13), 1, 8.
9 *W.N.M.A. Ann. Rep.* (1914), 2, 15.
10 *Report of the Committee of Inquiry into the anti tuberculosis service in Wales and Monmouthshire* (1939). H.M.S.O., London, p. 10.
11 *W.N.M.A. Ann. Rep.* (1910–13), 1, 9.
12 *Ibid.* (1914), 2, 167.
13 *Ibid.* (1910–13), 1, 20.
14 *Ibid.* (1914) 2, 18.
15 *Ibid.* (1914), 2, 32.
16 *Ibid.* (1910–13), 1, 19.
17 *Ibid.* (1914), 2, 124.
18 *Ibid.* (1914), 2, 44.
19 *Ibid.* (1914), 2, 46.
20 *Ibid.* (1914), 2, 163.

21 *Ibid.* (1910-13), 1, 51.
22 *Ibid.* (1918), 6, 9.
23 *Ibid.* (1917), 5, 12.
24 *Ibid.* (1915), 3, 36.
25 *Ibid.* (1918), 6, 5.
26 *Ibid.* (1916), 4, 25.
27 *Ibid.* (1914), 2, 39.
28 *Ibid.* (1917), 5, President's address.
29 *Ibid.* (1914), 2, 37.
30 *Ibid.* (1914), 2, 40.
31 *Ibid.* (1915), 3, 40.
32 *Ibid.* (1920), 8, 8.
33 *Ibid.* (1921), 9, 15.
34 *Ibid.* (1921), 9, 9.
35 *Ibid.* (1932), 20, 7.
36 *Ibid.* (1924), 12, 30.
37 *Ibid.* (1923), 11, 14.
38 *Ibid.* (1929), 17, 125.
39 *Ibid.* (1924), 12, 31.
40 *Ibid.* (1926), 14, 62.
41 *Ibid.* (1926), 14, 35.
42 *Ibid.* (1926), 14, 61.
43 *Ibid.* (1925), 13, 53.
44 *Ibid.* (1929), 17, 123.
45 *Ibid.* (1922), 10, 28.
46 *Ibid.* (1923), 11, 28.
47 *Ibid.* (1924), 12, 33.
48 *Ibid.* (1930), 18, 143.
49 *Ibid.* (1931), 19, 147.
50 *Ibid.* (1936), 24, 188.
51 *Ibid.* (1936), 24, 194.
52 *Ibid.* (1924), 12, 40.
53 *Ibid.* (1925), 13, 35.
54 *Ibid.* (1925), 13, 41.
55 *Ibid.* (1928), 16, 53.
56 *Ibid.* (1929), 17, 60.
57 *Ibid.* (1929), 17, 129.
58 *Ibid.* (1930), 18, 158.
59 *Ibid.* (1932), 20, 57.
60 *Ibid.* (1933), 21, 23.
61 *Ibid.* (1926), 14, 12.
62 *Ibid.* (1928), 16, 23.
63 *Ibid.* (1923), 11, 26.
64 *Ibid.* (1928), 16, 50.
65 *Ibid.* (1932), 20, 29.
66 *Ibid.* (1932), 20, 11.
67 *Ibid.* (1932), 20, 13.

68 *Ibid.* (1932), 20, 18.
69 *Ibid.* (1932), 20, back.
70 *King Edward VII Welsh National Memorial Association booklet.* Morgan, Laird & Co., Ltd., London, (c. 1932), 9.
71 *W.N.M.A. Ann. Rep.* (1936), 24, 36.
72 *Ibid.* (1937), 25, 137.
73 *Ibid.* (1937), 25, 32.
74 *Rep. Chf. Med. Offr. Minist. Hlth.* 1938 (1939), 143.
75 *W.N.M.A. Ann. Rep.* (1936), 24, 59.
76 *Ibid.* (1940), 28, 18.
77 *Ibid.* (1945), 33, 24.
78 *Ibid.* (1945), 33, 12.
79 *Ibid.* (1945), 33, 45.
80 *Ibid.* (1945), 33, 35.
81 *Ibid.* (1944), 32, 31.
82 *Ibid.* (1946), 34, 56.
83 *Ibid.* (1944), 32, 12.
84 *Ibid.* (1932), 20, 30.
85 *Ibid.* (1939), 27, 18.
86 *Ibid.* (1943), 31, 18.
87 *Ibid.* (1945), 33, 11.
88 *Ibid.* (1948), 36, 36.
89 *Ibid.* (1945), 33, 14.
90 *Ibid.* (1945), 33, 36.
91 *Ibid.* (1948), 36, 40.
92 *Rep. Welsh reg. Hosp. Bd. Tuberc. Serv.* (1948), 4.
93 *W.N.M.A. Ann. Rep.* (1947), 35, 11.
94 *Ibid.* (1944), 32, 18.
95 *Ibid.* (1948), 36, 11.
96 *Ibid.* (1946), 34, 34.

APPENDIX

RESEARCH PAPERS AND REPORTS PUBLISHED BY THE STAFF OF THE W.N.M.A., CONTAINED IN THE ANNUAL REPORTS

1 'Memorandum for the Guidance of Tuberculosis Physicians.' *W.N.M.A. Annual Report,* (1914), 2, 190.
2 Harries, E. H. R., 'Tuberculosis in Children'. *Ibid.* (1915), 3, 151.
3 'Report upon the Medical Policy of the Association'. *Ibid.* (1919), 7, 41.
4 Williams, T. G., 'Disinfection of Houses'. *Ibid.* (1919), 7, Appendix 1.
5 Thomas, J. L., 'Tuberculosis and the Garden City'. *Ibid.* (1928), 16, 142.
6 Thomas, M. P., 'Problem of the Ailing Child'. *Ibid.* (1928), 16, 143.
7 Watson, H. E., 'The Differential Diagnosis of Tuberculosis'. *Ibid.* (1928) 16, 145.
8 Williams, H. M., 'Pulmonary Tuberculosis in Children of School Age'. *Ibid.* (1928), 16, 147.

9 Clark, L. R., ' Synopsis of Cases Treated by Artificial Pneumothorax.' *Ibid.* (1929), 17, 123.
10 Rayner, A. E., ' The Importance of Radiography '. *Ibid.* (1929), 17, 125.
11 Ross, H. A., ' Breathing '. *Ibid.* (1929), 17, 126.
12 ' Investigation into the Radiological Appearances of the Chest in Coal Miners '. *Ibid.* (1929), 17, 129.
13 Lloyd, D. C., ' The High Mortality from Tuberculosis in Cardiganshire '. *Ibid.* (1930), 18, 143.
14 Matthews, R. J., ' The Aetiology of Tuberculosis '. *Ibid.* (1930), 18, 150.
15 Williams, H. M., ' Investigation on the Pirquet Test.' *Ibid.* (1930), 18, 153.
16 Jordan, N. T. K., ' Clinical Study on a Case of Tuberculosis, Silicosis and Anthracosis.' *Ibid.* (1930), 18, 156.
17 ' A radiological study of certain groups of "industrially healthy" South Wales Coal Miners '. *Ibid.* (1930), 18, 158.
18 Jones, V. E., ' An Analysis of Some of the End Results of Treatment of Tuberculosis in Anglesey '. *Ibid.* (1931), 19, 140.
19 Jones, D. W. F., ' Thoracoplastic Operations. (A record of cases treated at the North Wales Sanatorium up to March 31, 1931). *Ibid.* (1931), 19, 142.
20 Johnson, A. C. and Thomas, J. L., ' An Inquiry into the Incidence of Tuberculosis Occurring in the East Mon. Area During the Second Half of 1930. *Ibid.* (1931), 19, 147.
21 Williams, H. M., ' Boiler Scalers ' Lungs. *Ibid.* (1931), 19, 152.
22 Gilchrist, J. C., ' A Review of Some Recovered Cases, with Critical Notes on Diagnosis.' *Ibid* (1932), 20, 147.
23 Hiley, R. M., ' The Relation of Tuberculosis to Pregnancy, Parturition and the Puerperium '. *Ibid.* (1932), 20, 157.
24 Folliott, E., ' A short Analysis of Cases Under 15 years of Age, Admitted to Pontsarn Hospital from December 1914 to December 1931 '. *Ibid.* (1932), 20, 160.
25 Brownlee, A., ' Cases Illustrating the Differential Diagnosis of Tuberculosis.' *Ibid.* (1933), 21, 141.
26 Burns, C. W., ' The After-results of Surgical Patients Discharged from Kensington Hospital, St. Brides, between 1923 and 1927 '. *Ibid.* (1933), 21, 145.
27 Davies, T. W., ' Pulmonary Tuberculosis in Relation to Bone and Joint Tuberculosis '. *Ibid.* (1933), 21, 147.
28 Davies, W., ' Tuberculous Pericarditis and Artificial Pneumopericardium '. *Ibid.* (1933), 21, 149.
29 Ross, H. A., ' Epituberculosis '. *Ibid.* (1934), 22, 142.
30 Wells, F., ' Infected Milk, a Common Cause of Non-pulmonary Tuberculosis in Children '. *Ibid.* (1934), 22, 144.
31 Thomas, M. P., ' Miliary Tuberculosis at the Clinic '. *Ibid.* (1934), 22, 148.
32 Watson, H. E., ' Analysis of Cases Admitted to South Wales Sanatorium During 1933.' *Ibid.* (1934), 22, 150.
33 Prosser-Evans, R. G., ' Hydatid Disease of the Lung in a Child '. *Ibid* (1934), 22, 153.
34 Cummins, S. L., ' Epidemiological Enquiry Cards. ' *Ibid.* (1935), 23, 163.

35 Tytler, W. H., 'A Series of Intradermal Tuberculin Tests'. *Ibid.* (1935), 23, 176.
36 Jordan, N. T. K., 'A Comparison Between the Results of Intradermal Tuberculin and the X-ray Findings in a Series of 59 Boy-patients.' *Ibid.* (1935), 23, 178.
37 Rayner, A. E., 'A Survey of Three Years' Admissions into Meadowslea Hospital.' *Ibid.* (1935), 23, 181.
38 Clark, L. R., 'A General Survey of Non-pulmonary (Bones and Joints) Cases Treated at the Adelina Patti Hospital'. *Ibid.* (1935), 23, 184.
38 Williams, H. M., 'Pulmonary Fibrosis due to Syphilis' *Ibid.* (1935), 23, 186.
40 Tomley, J. E., 'An Analysis of Death from Tuberculosis in Wales and Monmouthshire' *Ibid.* (1935), 23, 189.
41 Jones, D. W. F., 'A Record of the End Results of Cases Admitted to the North Wales Sanatorium for Observation for Tuberculosis from April 1, 1927 to December 31, 1935' *Ibid.* (1936), 24, 170.
42 Aslett, E., 'Problems in Differential Diagnosis at a Tuberculosis Dispensary. *Ibid.* (1936), 24, 177.
43 Davies, J. K., 'Pulmonary Abscess'. *Ibid.* (1936), 24, 180.
44 Clark, L. R., 'A Long-standing case of Empyema Treated by Air-tight drainage'. *Ibid.* (1936), 24, 183.
45 Leishman, A., 'Effusions in Artificial Pneumothorax'. *Ibid.* (1936), 24, 184.
46 Jones, V. E., 'Notes on the Incidence of Tuberculosis in Anglesey'. *Ibid.* (1936), 24, 188.
47 Johnson, A. C., 'Reflections on Family Tuberculosis'. *Ibid.* (1936), 24, 191.
48 Hutchinson, E. C., 'Tuberculosis in a Welsh Country Parish'. *Ibid.* (1936), 24, 194.
49 Brownlee, A., 'The Problem of the Chronic Surgical Case'. *Ibid.* (1937), 25, 239.
50 Trail, H., 'Differential Diagnosis. P7(B)'. *Ibid.* (1937), 25, 242.
51 Gilchrist, J. C., 'Experientia Docet'. *Ibid.* (1937), 25, 249.
52 Jones, V. E., 'End Results of Sanatorium Treatment'. *Ibid.* (1937), 25, 255.
53 Hawkins, F. S., 'Osteochondritis'. *Ibid* (1938), 26, 218.
54 Jarman, T. F., 'The Treatment of Tuberculous Cervical Glands'. *Ibid.* (1938), 26, 227.
55 Jones, J. G., 'Pulmonary Tuberculosis in Colliery Workers'. *Ibid.* (1938), 26, 233.
56 Thomas, D. M. E., 'Six Cases of Extrapleural Pneumothorax'. *Ibid.* (1938), 26, 243.
57 Evans, R. G. P., 'A Survey'. *Ibid.* (1938), 26, 251.
58 Williams, H. M., 'Actinomycosis of Lung'. *Ibid.* (1939), 27, 251.
59 Milne, R. L., 'Pleural Effusions'. *Ibid.* (1939), 27, 257.
60 'Report of an Investigation into the Incidence of Tuberculosis in the County of Anglesey'. *Ibid.* (1939), 27, 271.

(Note : After 1939 original articles were submitted to current medical journals, such publications being noted by the Principal Medical Officer in his report to the W.N.M.A.)

MILESTONES IN THE HISTORY OF MINERAL DUST PNEUMOCONIOSES

E. Posner

Sub specie aeternitatis the documented history of pneumoconiosis in Wales is very short and practically confined to the 20th century. However in the course of the past 50 years or so Welsh doctors, or physicians working in Wales have contributed as much to the knowledge of the pneumoconioses as have workers over centuries in other lands.

One type of the pneumoconioses—silicosis—goes back far into the Paleolithic age, when men with their bare hands removed flints from riverbanks and afterwards shaped them into weapons and utensils. Their successors, Neolithic men, discovered that the freshly dug flint before losing its water was more pliable than the 'dead' flint found on the surface. Thus flint digging started and although we do not know anything about the mortality and morbidity in prehistoric flint diggers, we know a little about their linear descendants in Suffolk.

Until the beginning of this century the Suffolk flint diggers used iron picks of almost the same shape as the deer horns found in the skeleton hands of prehistoric flint miners of the same age. The modern flint miners and knappers showed a mortality from respiratory disease seven times higher than that of other men living in the same district (Collis 1919). By the time that their peculiar chest disease was finally explained in terms of silicosis and silico-tuberculosis—from which they had been dying for millenia—the industry employed only a few part-time workers. (Hunter 1955).

A similar but less known proof that recognition of a specific industrial lung disease often takes a very long time was only recently described from the Transkei. It had been known for many years that Bantu women often at an early age suffered from a 'cryptogenic,' progressive pulmonary fibrosis. Only seven years ago Palmer and

Daynes (1967) identified the disease as classical silicosis, resulting from grinding mealimeal between quartzite stones in the confined spaces of African huts.

From the time our ancestors settled in permanent habitats until the Industrial Revolution the documented history of the pneumoconioses relates almost exclusively to metal mining. Exceptions are the two Egyptian mummies whose lungs miraculously survived over 4,000 years, in which the paleopathologists Ruffer (1921) and Shaw (1938) found anthracotic lymph-nodes.

Between 4000 and 3000 B.C. the Egyptians established permanent mining settlements in Sinai and Nubia. They crowded into them slaves of the lowest order, convicts, prisoners of war and forced labourers with their families. Diodorus Siculus (quoted from Rosen 1943) described the prevailing conditions in the Egyptian mines: 'All those in mining are fettered, held at work day and night and young children make their way through the galleries and throw up with great toil the broken stones to the surface.'

In England 2000 years later the famous report on the children in mines (Parliamentary Papers 1842) contained illustrations of children underground which excellently fit Diodorus's verbal description. Some Victorian industrial pharaos riduculed the Report as being based on the evidence of artful boys and ignorant girls. (Hansard 1842).

Metal mining swiftly developed with Greek greatness and Roman conquests, but working conditions hardly improved for many centuries. Titus Carus Lucretius asked in his great work *De rerum natura*, 'Don't you see how underground work pales . . . and how it shortens life?'; and Justinian bluntly stated: 'To be condemned to the mines is nothing better than a death sentence'. (Quoted from Rosen, 1943).

The few ancient writers who comment on the occupational hazards of miners invariably mention their laboured breathing and the pallid colour of their faces. Whether their pallor was due to malnutrition, bad ventilation, ankylostomiasis or silicosis, or to all these factors, remains unknown. However as the miners extracted most metals from sandstone and granite matrices, they could hardly have failed to contract silicosis.

The fall of the Roman Empire was accompanied by a decline of the European metal mining industry. It emerged again in the 14th and

15th centuries, in Central Europe, especially in the long mountain range between Bohemia and Saxony, the *Erzgebirge.*

From the 16th century onwards the first monographs and leaflets dealing specifically with miners' diseases started to appear. Presumably Ulrich Ellenbog's (died 1499) treatise of the poisonous dusts and fumes, printed after his death in 1524, was the first of their kind. Ellenbog still stood firmly on Galenian ground and exhorted the miners to protect themselves against dust and fumes by profuse sweating and by drinking vermouth or wine.

George Bauer better known as Agricola (1499-1555) left us by far the most comprehensive account of mining and miners' diseases in the 16th century. Agricola was a renaissance man par excellence, physician, technologist, artist and politician. In the 12th volume of his monumental work *De Re Metallica* (1556) he commented on the increasing depth and consequent dryness and dustiness of the Bohemian and Saxonian mines and described in some detail the ' asthma, suppurating lesions and visible emaciations ' of many mine workers. He lamented the ' fate of miners' wives, some of whom had married seven husbands all of whom this terrible consumption had carried away to a premature death '. From his descriptions it is clear that he described not only silicosis and silico-tuberculosis, but also certainly lung cancer. Only in the last century it became known that the Joachimsthal and Annaberg mines which Agricola intimately knew, were heavily contaminated with radon gas. (Härting & Hesse 1879, Löwy 1929).

Philippus Theophrastus Bombastus von Hohenheim (1493-1541) who fortunately for posterity chose to be called simply Paracelsus had his magnum opus *Von der Bergsucht und Bergkrankheiten* (Miners' phthisis and miners' diseases) published posthumously in 1567. He clearly recognised the miners' phthisis as a specific occupational disease caused by noxious gases and dust. Paracelsus, a great iconoclast and vehement enemy of Galen and Avicenna had not quite thrown off the shackles of ancient and primitive magic medicine. He believed that the contamination of the air was ruled by astral constellations and that the miners' respiratory symptoms were due to sedimentation of tartarus in the airways—tartarus at that time meaning a mixture of salt, sulphur and mercury. He recommended washing it from the lungs by excessive sweating. For the prevention of miners' phthisis he prescribed :

Liquoris tartari unz.i.j.
Olei Colcotarini scrup.j.
Laudani purissimi drach. semis.

It is a sobering thought that up to our days clinical pharmacology had nothing more useful to offer in the field of the prevention and cure of pneumoconiosis.

Agricola's and Paracelsus' magna opera overshadowed a considerable number of highly interesting publications on mining diseases by contemporary minor authors, for which room cannot be found in this short paper.However, the Dutch anatomist and physician Diemerbroeck (1609-1674) must be honoured because he gave the first, accurate account of a dissected stone mason's lung and what is more, described what must be the first documented dust count : ' I know of a mason who hung up in his workshop a cattle bladder in which he found after one year a handful of dust, a quantity which leads to the death of the careless worker.' (1679)

Bernardo Ramazzini (1633-1714), who is rightly called the father of occupational medicine, embodied most of the contemporary knowledge on miners' diseases in his great work *De Morbis Artificum* (1700). He leaned heavily on Agricola and deplored conditions underground which had not materially changed since Roman times. Like most of those who wrote on miners' phthisis in the 18th century he was a pessimist in the field of therapy. ' Miners are liable to violent diseases which elude all manners of cure. Indeed it seems doubtful whether we ought to reckon it a pious office to prescribe physic to such wretches and thereby prolong their miserable life.' However he also wrote ' as great profits arise to princes and merchants from mines, and as the use of metals is highly necessary to almost all arts we are bound in duty to preserve the lives of these workmen by investigating their diseases.' Ramazzini's mercantilistic pronouncements show that the Industrial Revolution and early capitalism were already knocking at the door of the old society.

The predominant type of mineral dust pneumoconiosis during the Industrial Revolution and indeed until the 20th century was silicosis which haunted many manufactories—pottery, needle grinding cutlery production—to name only a few. Towards the end of the 19th century asbestos, the most dangerous dust of all, entered the scene, unnoticed until the 1930's. As my brief for this paper is ' Milestones in the History of Pneumoconiosis with particular reference to

Wales,' I must regretfully omit the story of the potters' rot, grinders' asthma, etc., and refer the reader to the excellent reviews by Holland 1843, Arlidge 1892, Hunter 1955 and Meiklejohn 1969.

Coalmining started in Britain in the 13th century on a rather small scale. Only when in the 16th century timber became scarce as a source of domestic heating, did it become a real industry. (Nef 1932).

In the first half of the 19th century the British coalmining industry employed 320,000 men, women and children. Employment of women and children was particularly rife in the Scottish coalfields. The previously quoted Parliamentary Report of 1842 bluntly stated : 'The seeds of painful and mortal disease are very often sown in childhood. Each generation of this class is commonly extinct soon after 50.'

At the beginning of the 19th century it had become evident that many miners suffered and died of the 'Black Lung' but great confusion reigned in respect of the origin and natural history of the disease. In France the great Laënnec—against vociferous opposition—attempted a clear definition between true 'melanosis' and the '*materière noire pulmonaire*,' found on the lung surfaces of city dwellers. He also observed in the lungs of coalminers masses resembling '*un morceau de savon noir*,' i.e. a piece of black soap which strongly suggests progressive massive fibrosis. Laënnec also tentatively suggested that the pulmonary black matter originated from the inhalation of smoke and soot (Laënnec 1826).

On the other hand in Germany the leader of German pathology R. Virchow (1847) denied the exogenous origin of the 'black lung' and proposed an endogenous process in the way of denaturation of small pulmonary haemorrhages caused by the heavy work and deep breathing of the colliers. Most German pathologists followed their master in this erroneous view.

Meanwhile in 1813 Dr C. Pearson read a paper on the 'Black spots in the lungs' to the Royal Society in London. The paper is a milestone as Pearson was convinced that coal dust enters the lungs on breathing, even if the dust is suspended in *invisible* particles.

From the 1830's onwards most relevant papers dealing with the miner's lung originated in Scotland. In 1831 J. C. Gregory published a 'Case of Peculiar Black Infiltration of the Lungs' in which he clearly stated that the diseases arose from coal mine dust. Another Scottish author, W. Marshall suggested that 'spurious melanosis' of the lungs was due to coalmine dust and not to the soot from miners' lamps.

In the first British monograph on industrial diseases Charles Thackrah Turner suggested that the pulmonary disease of miners was due to the inhalation of pyrites but he admitted that in some cases ' melanosis ' resembled or was identical with coal (1832).

Finally in 1838 Stratton cut through the Gordian knot of confusing nosology and proposed the name anthracosis for the coalminer's black lung, a term which became widely accepted.

In 1867 Zencker in Bavaria described a ' red lung ' of a woman who for many years had stained blotting paper with iron pigment. He coined the name ' siderosis ' and wrote the prophetic words : ' After we have learned to recognise anthracosis and siderosis, we may expect that other comparable diseases will be detected. It will be necessary to embrace under a single title all these essentially identical forms of the disease. The name PNEUMONOKONIOSIS recommends itself'. Visconti in 1870 added the term silicosis, which for many years was to overshadow the coalworker's black lung.

In the middle of the 19th century the foremost expert in the field of industrial dust disease was doubtlessly Dr Edward Headlam Greenhow, a medical officer on the staff of Sir John Simon. He visited all mining districts in England and Wales where an excessive amount of respiratory disease in miners had become known, consulted with mine owners and colliers and concluded in 1862 : ' Some miners retain their health till an advanced period of life but the greater number suffer, more or less from asthmatic symptoms before attaining the age of 50, and many break down and are disabled at from 40 to 50 years of age.'

Furthermore Greenhow suggested that the variety of diseases known as miners' phthisis, potters' rot, grinders' asthma etc., are all due to the inhalation of industrial dusts which cause interstitial pulmonary fibrosis.

After this the interest in anthracosis gradually faded out. The reason for this strange development—especially at a time of deepening mines and growing mechanisation—is still a matter of controversy. The fact is that most leading figures in Occupational Medicine considered the chapter of the ' black lung ' closed. Oliver in 1908 stated that the disease no longer existed in the British coalfields. In 1914 Shufflebotham declared in a Milroy lecture ' at present in Great Britain pulmonary fibrosis in miners is practically non existing ' and

Collis (1919) went even further by stating 'miners' asthma passed unobserved from our midst, and conjectures as to its character and causation are idle.' In the 1930's the highly influential physiologist J. S. Haldane violently battled against those who considered anthracosis as a specific and potentially disabling disease, a controversy which has been well described by Meiklejohn (1952). One must agree with Fletcher (1948) that these pronouncements by eminent men were largely responsible for the fact that mining engineers relaxed their efforts to reduce dust at a time of increasing mechanisation.

Inevitably in the 1920's anthracosis raised its head again and this time in Wales. By that time 30 years had passed since Röntgen had described his X-rays (1895), and slowly but steadily chest radiology had advanced to a point when it became possible to register not only large massive shadows, but also smaller opacities on the X-ray plate, Radiological evidence had become the most important factor in the triad of industrial history, clinical findings and X-rays in the diagnosis of specific dust disease. It was first used for field surveys in Australia (Gandevia 1973), and it noteworthy that as early as 1925 Nelson in Western Australia conducted a multidisciplinary survey of a mining population almost 20 years earlier than similar attempts were made in Britain.

Also in the early 20th century the medical staff of the South African Mining Bureau made outstanding contributions, in many aspects to the pneumoconiosis problem, especially the silicosis of gold-miners (Meiklejohn 1952, Orenstein, 1957).

By and large the central dogmata of pneumoconiosis research, i.e. 'Without free silica no silicosis' and 'Pneumoconiosis is synonymous with silicosis' remained intact until they were eventually shaken as the result of investigations in Wales. Tattersall wrote in 1926 from Wales, 'I was with increasing frequency encountering a disease which was either not tuberculous or—when proved to be tuberculous was of a type quite different in onset, course and X-ray findings from what one may call the straightforward case of tuberculosis'. In 1930 Cummins and Sladden maintained that in the anthracite miners in south Wales coal dust was capable of accumulating in the lungs and causing serious and fatal disease.

They still maintained that the presence of silica in the coalmine dust was a *conditio sine qua non* in causing anthracotic fibrosis. Collis and Gilchrist (1928) examined the coaltrimmers in south Wales ports and concluded that after a few years the lungs of coaltrimmers are not normal and exhibit signs similar to those widely regarded as characteristic of silicotic fibrosis. Whilst all this was said, until 1934 the right for claiming compensation remained confined to colliers engaged in drilling and blasting in siliceous rocks.

Then suddenly and as so often in the history of occupational disease without any hard and fast scientific evidence, the government of the day decided to include *all* underground workers into the (Various Industries) Silicosis Scheme. A veritable avalanche of claims followed especially from the anthracite mines near Swansea. The mine owners now contended that the chest disease of south Wales miners was pneumoconiosis and not silicosis and that *ergo ipso* the claimants were outside the compensation scheme. In this attitude they were aided by Haldane who attributed the miners' disease to tuberculosis, bronchitis and bronchiectasis. (McVittie 1949).

Between 1933 and 1935 the number of claims by miners—almost entirely from south Wales rose by 70 % and the high rate of refusals of certificates by the Silicosis Boards (McVittie 1953) clearly showed that the time had come for a major investigation of the characteristic X-ray appearances, pathological aspects and environmental conditions in the south Wales coalfields. The Medical Research Council entrusted Drs D'Arcy Hart and Aslett with the medical aspects of the problem. Their report (Privy Council, M.R.C. 1942) was published in the middle of the war and must be acclaimed as a major milestone, because it established the immensely important fact that coalminers' pneumoconiosis is a condition per se and different from classical silicosis.

They clearly showed that the X-rays of south Wales anthracite and steam coal miners showed a large proportion of radiological abnormalities not only in hard headers but also in coalface workers and other workmen underground. They considered the so-called ' reticulation as the earliest radiological sign of coalworkers' pneumoconiosis and thought it probable that reticulation can in a number of cases develop into gross fibrosis. With improved X-ray techniques the term reticulation has now become defunct. The reticular pattern was shown to be due to small coal nodules surrounded by focal emphysema. (Hepplestone 1951, Gough 1949).

Consequently the Committee on Industrial Pulmonary Disease

recommended the comprehensive term 'pneumoconiosis of coal-workers' for all pulmonary conditions described as due to dust in underground colliers, certain surface workers and coal trimmers. The committee also recommended that cases with reticulation should be taken into consideration for compensation purposes.

Perhaps the most important result of Hart's and Aslett's report was the setting up of a Pneumoconiosis Research Unit in Penarth, which has over the years become one of the main centres of pneumoconiosis research in the world. Many of the findings and hypotheses of the scientific workers of the P.R.U. are of recent date and must therefore await analysis and judgment by future historians. However, there are some achievements which certainly will stand the test of time :

1. Epidemiological surveys, based on a broad multidisciplinary approach and relating environmental measurements with biological responses, based on standardised radiographic, clinical and physiological examination and lung pathology. With regard to pathology the close co-operation with Prof. J. Gough and his team of the Welsh National School of Medicine cannot be over stated.

2. The drawing up of a logical scheme of radiological abnormalities thus allowing clinicians and research workers to compare their results on a national and international scale.

3. The correlation of radiological and physiological changes.

4. The epidemiological studies of whole industrial communities as the basis for studying the effect of specific exposures on morbidity and mortality.

5. The testing of the intra- and inter-observer error applied to radiology, clinical examination and physiology which had a most important effect on the reliability of statistical evaluations.

There are already signs that this intensive work of the past 25 years or so, combined with the excellent contributions by the Medical Officers of the National Coal Board has benefited not only the south Wales collier but dust exposed workers all over the world. There can be little doubt that the work done at the Pneumoconiosis Research

Unit and Cardiff Medical School will one day be assessed as one of the foremost contributions from Wales to the History of Medicine.

ACKNOWLEDGEMENTS:

I am greatly indebted to Miss M. Gregory, Librarian of the Pneumoconioses Research Unit at Penarth, to Mr P. J. Bishop, Librarian of the Cardio-Thoracic Institute in London and to Mrs R. Woosnam, Librarian of the North Staffs Medical Institute for providing me with documentary material for this paper. I also sincerely thank Mrs M. Hampton for secretarial help.

REFERENCES

Agricola, G. (1556). *De Re Metallica Libri XII.* Froben and Bischoff, Basle, (English translation by H. C. Hoover and L. H. Hoover, *Mining Magazine,* London, 1912).

Arlidge, J. T. (1892). *The Hygiene, Diseases and Mortality of Occupations.* Percival, London.

Collis, E. L. (1919). *Industrial Pneumoconioses, with Special Reference to Dust-Phthisis.* H.M.S.O., London.

Collis, E. L., and Gilchrist, J. C. (1928). Effects of dust upon coal trimmers. *J. Ind. Hyg.,* 10, 101.

Cummins, S. L., and Sladden, A. F. (1930). Coal-miner's lung : an investigation into the anthracotic lungs of coal-miners in S. Wales. *J. Path. Bact.,* 33, 1095.

Diemerbroeck, I. de. (1679) *Anatome Corporis Humani,* new ed. Huguetan, Lyons.

Diodorus Siculus (Ist cent. B.C.) Quoted from Rosen (1943) pp. 12-14.

Ellenbog, U. (1524). *Von den gifftigen Besen Tempffen und Reüchen der Metal, etc.* Augsburg. (Facsimile ed., Munich, 1927. English translation, *Lancet,* 1, 270, 1932).

Fletcher, C. M. (1948). Pneumoconiosis of coal-miners. *Br. med. J.,* 1, 1015 and 1065.

Gandevia, B. (1973). The Australian contribution to the history of the pneumoconioses. *Med. Hist.,* 17, 368

Gough, J. (1949). The pathology of pneumoconiosis. *Postgrad. med. J.,* 25, 611.

Greenhow, E. H. (1862). *Fourth Report of the Medical Officer of the Privy Council* 1861, p. 138, Appendix IV. H.M.S.O., London (quoted from Meiklejohn 1951).

Gregory, J. C. (1831). Case of peculiar black infiltration of the whole lungs, resembling melanosis. *Edinb. med. surg. J.,* 36, 389.

Hansard, House of Lords (1842). June 24th.

Härting, F. H., and Hesse, W. (1879). Der Lungenkrebs, die Bergkrankheit in den Schneeberger Gruben. *Vischr. gericht. Med. öff. Sanitwes.*, 30, 296; 31, 102 and 313.

Hepplestone, A. G. H. (1951). Coal workers' pneumoconiosis. *A.M.A. Archs. ind. Hyg.*, 4, 270.

Holland, G. C. (1843) *Diseases of the Lungs from Mechanical Causes.* Churchill, London.

Hunter, D. (1955). *The Diseases of Occupations,* 1st ed. English Universities Press, London.

Laënnec, R. T. H. (1826). *Traité de l'Anscultation Médiate,* 2nd ed. Chaudé, Paris.

Lucretius, Titus Carus (1st cent. B.C.) *De Rerum Natura Libri VI.*

McVittie, J. C. (1949) Pneumoconiosis in coal miners. *Postgrad. med. J.*, 25, 186.

McVittie, J. C. (1953) In *Proceedings of the Third International Conference of Experts on Pneumoconiosis: Sydney:* 1950, Vol. 1, p. 172. International Labour Office, Geneva.

Löwy, J. (1929). Uber die Joachimstaler Bergkrankheit *Med. Klin.*, 25, 141.

Marshall, W. (1833-34). Cases of spurious melanosis of the lungs or of phthisis melanotica. *Lancet*, 2, 271.

Medical Research Council (1942). Chronic pulmonary disease in S. Wales coalminers. I. Medical studies. (B. Medical survey, by P. D'Arcy Hart and E. A. Aslett). *Spec. Rep. Ser. med. Res. Coun.*, 243.

Meiklejohn, A. (1951). History of lung diseases of coal miners in Great Britain. Part I. *Br. J. ind. Med.*, 8, 127.

Meiklejohn, A. (1952). History of lung diseases of coal miners in Great Britain. Part III. *Br. J. ind. Med.*, 9, 208.

Meiklejohn, A. (1969). The history of occupational respiratory disease in the North Staffs. pottery industry. In *Health Conditions in the Ceramic Industry,* ed. by C. N. Davies, p. 3. Pergamon Press, Oxford.

Nef, J. U. (1932). *The Rise of the British Coal Industry.* Routledge, London.

Nelson, W. T. (1926). *Report on an Investigation of the Pulmonary Condition of Mine Employees of W. Australia.* Service Publ. No. V, Div. Indust. Hyg., Canberra.

Oliver, T. (1908). *Diseases of Occupations.* Methuen, London.

Orenstein, A. J. (1957). The history of pneumoconiosis. *S. Afr. med. J.*, 31, 797.

Palmer, P. E. S., and Daynes, G. (1967). Transkei silicosis. *S. Afr. med. J.*, 41, 1182.

Paracelsus [Theophrastus Bombastus von Hohenheim] (1567). *Von der Bergsucht oder Bergkranckheiten.* Mayer, Dillingen.

Parliamentary Papers (1842). XV-XII. Quoted from Pike, E. R. (1966). *Human Documents of the Industrial Revolution.* Allen and Unwin, London.

Pearson, G. (1813). On the colouring matter of the black bronchial glands and of the black spots in the lungs. *Phil. Trans. R. Soc.*, 103, 159.

Privy Council, Medical Research Council (1942) Spec. Report Series. No. 243. *Chronic Pulmonary Disease in South Wales Coalminers.* Part B. Medical Survey by P. D' Arcy Hart and E. A. Aslett with contributions by D. Hicks and R. Yates. Part C. Pathological Report by T. H. Belt and A. A. Ferris. London, H.M.S.O.

Ramazzini, B. (1700). *De Morbis Artificum Diatriba.* Capponi, Modena.

Röntgen, W. C. (1895). Ueber eine neue Art von Strahlen. Sber. phys.—med. Ges. Würzb., 29, 132. (Facsimile *Isis,* 26, 365, 1937).

Rosen, G. (1943). *The History of Miners' Diseases.* Schuman, New York.

Ruffer, M.A. (1921). *Studies in the Paleopathology of Egypt,* p. 15. University of Chicago Press, Chicago.

Shaw, A. F. B. (1938) A histological study of the mummy of Har-Mose, the singer of the 18th dynasty. *J. Path. Bact.,* 47, 115.

Shufflebotham, F. (1914). The hygienic aspect of the coal-mining industry in the United Kingdom III. Br. *med. J.,* 1, 588.

Silius, Italicus (1st cent. A.D.) Quoted from Rosen (1943), p. 36.

Stratton, T. (1838) Case of anthracosis or black infiltration of the whole lungs. *Edinb. med. surg. J.,* 49, 490.

Tattersall, N. (1926). The occurrence and clinical manifestations of silicosis among hard ground workers in coal mines. *J. ind. Hyg. Toxicol.,* 8, 466.

Thackrah, C. T. (1832) *The Effects of Arts, Trades, and Professions,* 2nd ed. Longman, London.

Virchow, R. (1847). Die pathologischen Pigmente. *Virchows Arch. path. Anat. Physiol.,* 1, 434 and 461.

Visconti, L. (1870). *Protocollo Generale delle Necropsie Seguite nell' Istituto Anatomo Patologico dell' Ospedale Maggiore.*

Zenker, F. A. (1867). Ueber Staubinhalationskrankheiten der Lungen, *Dt. Arch. Klin. Med.,* 2, 116.

THE HISTORY OF COAL MINERS' SKIN DISEASES

GEOFFREY A. HODGSON

Ramazzini (1746) made the fundamental distinction 'that the various and manifold diseases which attacked workers sprung from two main causes,' the first being the harmful characters of the materials handled and the second the violent and irregular motions and unnatural positions of the body by which the natural structure of the vital machine is impaired. This is particularly true of coal miners, whose skin disorders have been directly related to the progressive changes in mining technology from the earliest times to the present day. The story of the Welsh coal mines is representative of mining throughout Britain.

Possibly coal was used by ancient Britons ; a prehistoric flint axe has been found in a coal outcrop at Craig y Parc (Evans 1961). The earliest miners in Wales may have been monks of the Cistercian monastery at Margam, Glamorgan nearby the present Port Talbot steel works. They mined at Felinfach near Llanfabon in 1284 (Evans 1961), the coal being used for lime burning, the smithy and malting.

The first mines were shallow excavated pits called bell pits. During the fourteenth and fifteenth centuries the room and pillar method developed. The bell pits were made square, like adjacent cells in a honeycomb, forming rooms with coal pillar walls. Methods described by Dr George Bauer (1494-1555), known as Agricola (1556) and Philippus Theophrastus Bombastus von Hohenheim (1493-1541) known as Paracelsus in the metal and coal mines of Bohemia, were representative of those used in mediaeval mines in Britain. Men entered the mine either by a basket, straddling a wooden horse, or holding a rope with one leg through it.

By the sixteenth century mining in Britain had become commonplace, most of the pits being either open cast or bell pits in surface seams. In Pembroke, George Owen of Henllys (1552-1613) describes how the early room and pillar pits sunk six or seven foot square, had a windlass turned by four men drawing the coal through the ' down-right ' door. Later pits were twelve to twenty fathoms deep with sundry holes for two, three or four men. Each man had a candle, ' Sitting as he worketh '. Stooping boys carried a loaded basket on their backs to the door, where it was lifted up, returning with an empty one, (Lloyd & Lloyd 1969). Tools were pickaxes and hammers, with wedges and fledges to break the coal.

During the seventeenth century the removal of the coal walls wastefully left behind in the pillar and room method, led to the long wall technique. The coal face was mined throughout its length, the roof being supported by rubble behind, with timber pit props in front. Coal was exported from south Wales to Ireland and Cornwall for tin smelting and to north Wales for lead and sulphur smelting (Evans 1961). As pits became deeper, the problems of ventilation, lighting and flooding became more difficult.

Drainage was improved by steam engines, such as Thomas Savory's ' miners' friend ' (1768) and James Watt's engine (1769). But ventilation was primitive as few pits had two shafts, and miners choking from black damp vainly swung their coats ' to and fro '. Gun powder inserted in a leather bag, first used in Britain in 1670 for blasting (Rosen 1943) increased explosions from fire damp (methane).

Miners attributed falls to demons who pushed them down or put out their lights by chattering. In Wales noises from earth movements were accepted as ill omens well into the nineteenth century. Very bad were whistlings and the *tolaeth* with shuffling and trampling noises suggesting people carrying coffins. The ' knockers ' were friendly fairy creatures however who pointed to the best seams (Davies 1972).

Legislation protected the coal owner and his mines, rather than the health of the workers.

EIGHTEENTH CENTURY

The finding of iron ore, and limestone for steel working led to rapid expansion of coal mining in Wales. By 1750 there were seven blast furnaces in south Wales and twenty-six by 1796. Famous names include John Maybury at Hirwaun (1759) and Thomas Guest at Merthyr (1793) The building of canals and railways followed. A few pits got much deeper, down to 600 feet at Bryncoch (Evans 1961). Labour flooded into Wales from Ireland and England.

Most coal was still won by pick and shovel, and haulage done by men or women carrying baskets or pushing wheel barrows. Pit ponies were not taken underground till 1750 (Rosen 1943). Up and down shafts improved ventilation, with air flow directed by partitions or trap doors. Lighting methods included candles, lanterns and steel mills producing sparks. Whilst even sunlight reflected by mirrors was used as in the tombs of ancient Egypt.

Pockets of fire damp were deliberately exploded by a fireman in old wet clothes, who lay face downwards with a light on the end of a long stick.

NINETEENTH CENTURY

The pits became still deeper. Advances in technology included exhaust fans and Davy's safety lamp devised at the request of the Rev. John Hodgson's Sunderland Society, formed to prevent mine accidents. Double deck cages and wire ropes with stronger steam engines improved haulage, but even in 1840 Pembroke women, in groups of six, still worked windlasses to wind the baskets up the shaft (Evans 1972). Labour was hired in gangs with a charter master 'gaffer' or 'contractor' as an intermediary between the mine owner and the men. Piece-work wages were paid in pubs often owned by the 'butty'.

Brick houses with three to four rooms were built in drab rows on the hillsides. Each had furniture, a Welsh testament, a clock on the wall, a good side of bacon and a bag of herbs, but no drainage and few if any privies (Morris & Williams 1958). Work clothes were dried before the fire. A tub bath was taken once a week, the centre of the back being left unwashed, in case it was weakened. Welsh rugby players and boxers were to be recognised by their blackened spines for many years to come. Strikes, with riots, came from attempts to reduce wages or when 'foreign' labour tried to enter the pits. A twelve hour day was usual. Young children were air door openers, carters dragging skips by a chain fixed to a leather girdle, whilst older boys pushed coal trams or led horses (Evans 1972). Colliers bought candles and gun powder out of their own wages. Seams were so low that men near naked worked sitting or reclining (Rosen 1943).

LABOUR LEGISLATION

The first Factory Act after a bitter struggle had been passed in 1833.

It was however the appalling working conditions of the children of the poorer classes in the mines and elsewhere, brought to light by the enquiry of Lord Ashley (Earl of Shaftesbury), which prompted the 1842 Act. This was a landmark in limiting the employment of women and children in the mines. Next, public concern about the frequent explosions and the reports of the social conditions of miners by the first appointed commissioner Mr Tremenheere led to the Act for mines inspection in 1850. Inspectors were appointed. By 1872 the Coal Mines Regulation Act had begun to approximate lighting, ventilation, explosives, etc. to the requirements of present day legislation. In the same year the compulsory education of children under 13 virtually put a stop to the employment of young persons. Further acts on explosives, dust suppression, rescue (1887-1911 and since) have amended the regulations.

These early acts paved the way for scientific research into technology and later legislation demanded recognition of occupational skin disease.

SCIENTIFIC AND TECHNICAL RESEARCH

Prevention of explosions became a prime concern. During 1851—1855 there had been 738 deaths in south Wales, one fifth involving boys who fell in front of the trams (Morris & Williams 1958).

It had been noted by John Buddle in 1803 that persons could be burned by sparks at a distance after an explosion, which did not occur on roads with unburnable ash. Coal dust was incriminated in the 1879 report of the Royal Commission, and after successful tests, stone dusting became statutory in 1920. In most years before this, such as those between 1880—1910, explosions killed some 1000—1500 miners in British pits (Arnot 1953). Major Welsh disasters in 1880 occurred at Risca (120 killed) and at the Naval Steam Colliery, Glamorgan (101 killed).

Dust suppression by water infusion arose from the 1911 Act recommending cleansing the roads with water. Silicosis was by then recognised. But two years later in 1913 an appalling explosion at Senghenydd killed 439 men. Other measures for dust suppression included Salt (1906) and Calcium Chloride (1938).

TWENTIETH CENTURY

In 1901 only 1.5% of all coal was extracted by mechanisation. By 1913 it rose to 7.7% with over a million (1,107,000) miners employed. Whilst by 1938 mechanisation was responsible for 59% but with now a labour force of three quarters of a million (Arnot 1953). Automatic picks began to replace the mandril, and oil-filled hydraulic hand operated Dowty props (1945) were used as roof supports instead of timber.

Today's machines such as the Anderton-Shearer were introduced in 1953-55 (Brown 1973) and since 1966 rotating toothed-cylinder trepanners have cut the whole face, with automatic powered face supports behind. Armoured conveyors with belts transported coal to the surface. So that by 1965 there were only 485,000 miners left. In 1972 the labour force was 280,000, which is still contracting. In comparison the 70,000 pit ponies of 50 years ago have decreased to 600 in 1971 (Report 1972).

HEALTH LEGISLATION AND MEDICAL CARE

Before 1842 medical care of miners was given by 'truck doctors' paid from the men's wages. Each was responsible for 15,000 miners or 20,000 if they had an unqualified assistant. Later it was taken over by general practitioners on contract.

Lord Campbell's Fatal Accident Act 1846 had allowed near relations to claim (Arnot 1953) after the death of a miner. Legislation allowing compensation for industrial accidents came later and for designated occupational diseases only in the present century. The first medical inspector of mines, appointed in 1924 to deal with first aid and ambulance services, joined the inspectorate in 1927.

Only six scheduled diseases for compensation were designated in the Workmen's Compensation Act 1906. Others were later added and became 'Prescribed diseases' (PD) under the National Health (Industrial Injuries) Act 1946.

The National Health Act came in 1948 and a colliery medical service under the Chief Medical Officer of the National Coal Board in 1947.

OCCUPATIONAL SKIN DISORDERS

As Sand (1952) remarks 'a new disease however is a rare thing and all we do now is to categorise them with greater accuracy than before '. It is convenient to discuss miners' disorders in two groups :

(*a*) Industrial Injuries (Accidents)

(*b*) Prescribed diseases (scheduled occupational skin disorders).

(*a*) *Industrial Injuries* (*Accidents*)

Wounds from explosions and falls of ground have always been common. Abrasions, common today, were also common in boys who scraped themselves against the wall as they clung to the basket, not being allowed inside it with the men (Evans 1972). Colliery log books recall many skin injuries in 1860 from ' blowers ' and falls (Morris & Williams 1958). There were no first aid boxes. Dust in an eye was removed by a man's tongue, cobwebs stopped bleeding, pit prop gum was used on open wounds, and tram grease, bacon fat and tea leaves on burns, or the part soaked in oil or paraffin was further exposed to close heat from a fire (Davies 1972). Two skin disorders are accepted as industrial accidents under the Industrial Injuries Act (1946).

(i) *Disfiguring Scars*

Coal dust penetrating a wound causes anthracotic tattoos. Noted by Fabry & Bockhold (1926) these pigmented scars or ' colliers stripes ' (Bettley 1940) are occupational stigmata also mentioned by Prosser White (1915) in Britain. Blast injury from burst compressed air pipes cause greater disfigurements today.

(ii) *Dermatophytosis*

The first pithead baths in Wales were installed at North Celynen Colliery in 1932.

Where pithead baths are used, tinea pedis (athletes foot) can be accepted as an industrial accident since the commissioner in 1949 (Commissioners decision 1949) upheld the decision of a local appeal tribunal in favour of a claimant. He said, 'there is a strong inference that the disease was caused by the ' bacilli ' (*sic*) of epidermophytosis which are present at the pithead baths '. In fact the fungi Trichophyton Interdigitale and T. rubrum are more commonly found (English 1957). The commission's decision has been supported in practice by Gentles & Holmes (1957) in Britain who found 31 % of miners using the baths to be infected with tinea pedis compared with 8 % of those who did not.

Foot ringworm in miners is still an important disease which in 1969-70 made up 3,160 of the 3,280 claims for injury benefit over all industry.

(b) Prescribed Diseases

Of the present total of forty-seven disorders scheduled under the Act as prescribed diseases, nine refer to coal miners (Fig. 1). Pneumoconiosis is prescribed, but not actually listed. The main skin disorders and their relation to changing mine environment and technology are discussed below.

Fig. 1

PRESCRIBED DISEASES (PD) IN COAL MINERS (1973)

P.D.	(17	Poisoning by Nitrous Fumes)
	21 (a)	Leptospirosis Icterohaemorrhagicae
	22	Ankylostomiasis (Hookworm)
	31	' Beat ' hand (Cellulitis)
	32	' Beat ' knee (Bursitis and Cellulitis)
	33	' Beat ' elbow (Bursitis and Cellulitis)
	34	Tenosynovitis
	(35	Miners' Nystagmus)
	42	Non-infective dermatitis of external origin (including chrome ulceration of the skin but excluding dermatitis due to ionising radiations other than radiant heat).

Leptospirosis (P.D. 21) (Leptospiral jaundice)

Leptospirosis is now divided into 21 (a) L. icterohaemorrhagicae ' work in places which are or are liable to be infested by rats ' and 21 (b) L. canicola from dogs. Infections come from rats which feed on scraps of food or pit ponies' fodder and possibly enter through abrasions or beat knee (Fisher 1944). Infections were notified in 1924 in Scottish coal mines (Report 1934). It was first listed in the Workmen's Compensation Act of 1940. During 1969—1972 in Britain only eleven cases were certified in all industry and none of these were in coal miners (Report 1971-72) because of effective rodenticides.

Ankylostomiasis (P.D. 22) (Hookworm)

Eggs of this intestinal parasite when excreted contaminate wet ground and the larvae cause ' ground itch ', with their burrowing of the feet of miners in warm climates. The anaemia and abdominal symptoms of seventeenth century miners, recorded by Ramazzini, suggest ankylostomiasis. Infections have been lessened with improved public health measures, but have continued in Germany up to the end of the last century with 1,355 cases in Bonn by 1902 (Report 1934). It was considered that the communal plunge propagated the infection, so individual shower baths were recommended.

At the end of the nineteenth century some Cornish tin mine workers were infected and in 1906 the Miners Federation asked the Home Office to appoint a commission, on which Dr J. S. Haldane served, to consider not only physical safety measures in coal mines such as watering the roads, lamps, etc., but also health hazards like ankylostomiasis. This was a scheduled miners' disease in the Workmen's Compensation Act of 1906. By the twenties, Prosser White (1928) considered Britain was quite exempt. Today it is an unlikely risk unless brought in again by immigrants.

' Beat ' conditions (P.D. 31, 32 & 33)

' Beat ' conditions comprised cellulitis of the hand (P.D. 31), and subcutaneous cellulitis of the knee (P.D. 32) or of the elbow (P.D. 33). First listed in 1907 ' simply to mining ', they now apply to all manual work. By 1919-23 ' beat ' knee became the second most common occupational disorder in miners after nystagmus. The rising incidence especially in Wales promoted an investigation by the Medical Research Council. Drs Collis and Llewellyn (1924) concluded that the cause was always repeated trauma from crawling or kneeling in thin seams, and hand damage from manual work. The average depth of seams in Britain for decades has been about 1.25 metres (4 feet). (Report 1970-71). They recommended the abolition of garters below the knee, the wearing of knee pads and smoothing of pick handles. The older collier having learned that he could harden his hands by urine in the pit or in the chamber pot at night (Davies 1972), was using a forerunner of the urea used in hand creams today. ' Beat ' knee is related to seam height (Watkins, Hunt, Fernandez & Edmonds 1958),—the pressure causing haemorrhages from sharp particles with the entry of staphylococcal infection (Atkins & Marks 1952). Modern pads cushion the knee, correcting extreme variations of pressure (Sharrard 1965). Although most 'beat' conditions are lessening in numbers due to mechanisation and better protection, 'beat' knee is still a problem in miners as kneeling is still necessary.

Tenosynovitis (P.D. 34)

First scheduled in 1906 'Traumatic inflammations of the hand or forearm tendons or of associated tendon sheaths' from repetitive manual work affects all manual workers. Mechanisation has but halved the rate in miners since 1951 (Report 1971-72).

Non-infective dermatitis (P.D. 42)

This was first scheduled in the Compensation Act 1906. Later it became P.D. 26 as an eczematous inflammation produced by dust or caustic or corrosive and now P.D. 42. Today in Britain the national average of spells of incapacity for Dermatitis (P.D. 42) is 0.8 per 1,000 (Newhouse 1972). Coal mining tops the list of industries having an incidence above the average (fig. 2).

Fig. 2 (Newhouse 1972)

HIGH RISK INDUSTRY RESPONSIBLE FOR P.D. 42 (1971) CLAIMS

Coal mining	4.6 per 1000 claims
Leather (including dyeing)	2.42
Metal goods	1.79
Chemicals	1.54
Metallurgy (oils)	1.25
Food and drink	1.3
Textiles	0.93

The term eczema is used here to include all eczematous inflammations for which injury benefit is paid under P.D. 42. Most eczemas in miners start on the feet and lower legs, and next on the hands and forearms (Rook & Hodgson 1956), (Hodgson 1955), (Matthews 1959), in contrast to other industries where the hands are first affected. Other specific patterns in miners are eczemas under the cap band, on the feet, under the belt or lamp battery, and under knee pads.

The predominance of P.D. 42 in miners has only emerged in the last two decades. References to eczema before this are rare in colliers in any textbooks.

Agricola (Sand 1952) writes of miners wearing gaiters for protection against stagnant cold water ' which is very bad for the nerves ' of the legs and Ramazzini (1746) of ulcerated legs ' apt to be vitiated in water '. Agricola had advised miners to wear rawhide boots because of the water, and gloves to the elbow (Teleky 1948). Lord Shaftesbury's Commission, before the 1842 Act, described the sore feet and legs swollen with boils, in children of five or six years standing in salty water (Wilson & Levy 1939). Willan (1808) described the first trade skin inflammations in bakers, cleaning women and masons. Tilbury Fox (1873) wrote of similar trade eczemas. Thackrah (1832) noted the sallow complexion, curved spines and the half-closed eyes from the coal dust irritated eyelids of colliers.

In the later nineteenth century skin disorders were considered unusual in Belgian miners (Böens-Boissau 1862) whilst the report of the Mines Commission of 1864 disregards them entirely (Report 1865). In other nineteenth and even in twentieth century articles on diseases of miners, references are still scanty. Up to the Second World War there are few reports of miners' eczema or other skin diseases. Occasional irritations such as ' water itch ' from mine water, intertrigo and dermatitis from creosoted props are recorded as specific miners' skin diseases by the International Labour Office in Geneva (Report 1934). But considering the environmental conditions and the low seams of the eighteenth and nineteenth century working, the absence of eczema seems remarkable. Even the classic textbook on industrial skin disorder of Prosser White (1915) does not mention eczema in coal miners and only irritation of the ears by coal dust is recorded in the American textbook (Schwartz, Tulipan & Peck 1947).

Miners' eczema which appears first to have been recognised in the early compensation acts, has grown to its present prominence only with National Insurance and the Industrial Injuries (1946) Act. It is usually a ' wear and tear ' eczema seen in the older man who has worked for over fifteen years (Sneddon 1951). Irritations come from frictional trauma in awkward seams, from clothes and equipment soiled by coal and stone dust or skin wetted by dust suppressant infusion and minewater.

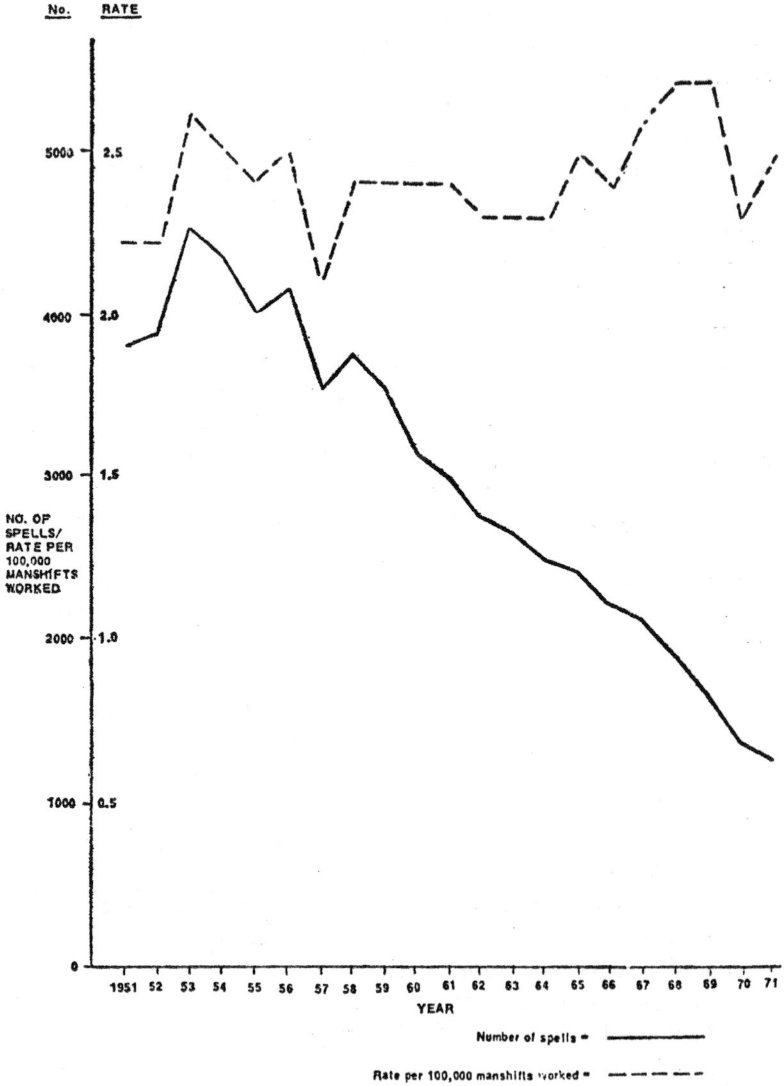

Fig. 3

NEW SPELLS OF INCAPACITY FROM DERMATITIS (P.D. 42)
1951—1971
(Annual Report NCB 1971-72)

Milarias, but rarely seen in British pits (Dowling & Brain 1934) are likely in deep hotter pits. Calcium chloride may cause necroses and calcinosis. (Zackheim and Pinkus). Contact acid burns from lamp batteries used to occur. Contact allergies are uncommon and where they occur reflect new mining technology such as hydraulic oils with special additives, rubber and plastics, cements, (chromate) explosive and medicaments from the first aid room used for injuries (Williamson & Vickers 1972).

In contrast to all the other prescribed diseases, spells of incapacity from P.D. 42 have not lessened in the last twenty years. Fig. 3 shows new spells of absence attributed to dermatitis 1951-71 and the rate per 100,000 manshifts worked.

These figures may not accurately indicate the prevalence of occupational eczema in miners. Matthews (1959) found that the incidence of constitutional eczema and miners' eczema to be about the same, both in a high claim (8 per 1000) and a low claim (4 per 1000) mine, but the fact remains that eczema remains a major cause of incapacity in coal miners.

REFERENCES

Agricola, G. (1556). *De Re Metallica Libri XII.* Froben and Bischoff, Basle (English translation by H. C. Hoover and L. H. Hoover. *Mining Magazine,* London, 1912).

Atkins, J. B., and Marks, J. (1952). *Br. J. Ind. Med.,* 9, 296.

Arnot, R. P. (1953). *The Miners : Years of Struggle.* Allen and Unwin, London.

Bettley, F. R. (1940). *Br. J. Derm.,* 52, 129.

Boëns—Boissau, H. (1862). *Traité Pratique des Maladies, des Accidents et des Difformités des Houilleurs.* Tircher, Brussels.

Brown, G. N. (1973). Personal communication.

Collis, E. L., and Llewellyn, T. L. (1924). *Spec. Rep. Ser. med. Res. Coun.,* 89.

Commissioners decision (1949). Ministry of National Insurance, National Insurance Act Claim for Industrial Injury benefit. C.I. 211/49 (KL) dated 7 Nov. 1949.

Davies, L. (1972). *Aspects of Mining Folklore in Wales,* reprinted from *Folk Life* National Museum of Wales, Cardiff.

Dowling, G. B., and Brain, R. T. (1934). *Br. J. Derm.,* 46, 215.

English, M. P. (1957). *Br. med. J.,* 1, 744.

Evans, E. W. (1961). *The Miners of South Wales.* University of Wales Press, Cardiff.

Evans, R. M. (1972). *Children in the Mines.* (1840–1842). Museum Schools Service. National Museum of Wales, Cardiff.

Fabry, J., and Bockholt, H. (1926). In *Die Schädigungen der Haut durch Beruf und gewerbliche Arbeit,* edited by K. Ullmann, M. Oppenheim, and J. H. Rille, Vol. 2, p. 285. Voss, Leipzig.

Fisher, S. W. (1944). *Br. J. ind. Med.,* 1, 153.

Fox, W. T. (1873). *Skin Diseases,* 3rd ed. Renshaw, London.

Gentles, J. C., and Holmes, J. G. (1957). *Br. J. ind. Med.,* 14, 22.

Hodgson, G. (1955). *Br. J. Derm.,* 67, 426.

Lloyd, D. M., and Lloyd, E. M. (1969). *A Book of Wales,* p. 168. Collins, London.

Matthews, B. F. (1959). *Br. J. ind. Med.,* 16, 200.

Morris, J. H., and Williams, L. J. (1958). *The South Wales Coal Industry* (1841–1875). University of Wales Press, Cardiff.

Newhouse, M. L. (1972). *Trans. a Rep. St. John's Hosp. derm. Soc. Lond.,* 58, 48.

Ramazzini, B. (1746). *A Treatise of the Diseases of Teadesmen.* London.

Report (1865). Report of Mines Commission, 1864. (Summary.) *Br. for. med. chir. Rev.,* 35, 361.

Report (1934). Report No. 68. ' Occupation and Health ', Industrial Labour Office, Geneva.

Report (1971/72). *Annual Report, National Coal Board,* Supplement. *The Prescribed Diseases of Coal Miners other than Pneumoconiosis.* H.M.S.O., London.

Report (1972). *Black Diamonds : silver anniversary National Coal Board,* 1947—1972.

Rook, A., and Hodgson, G. (1956). *Br. J. Ind. Med.*, 13, 281.
Rosen, G. (1943). *The History of Miners' Diseases.* Schuman, New York.
Sand, R. (1952). *The Advance to Social Medicine.* Staples Press, London.
Schwartz, L., Tulipan, L., and Peck, S. M. (1947). *Occupational Diseases of the Skin.* Henry Kimpton, London.
Sharrard, W. J. W. (1965). *Ann. R. Coll. Surg.*, 36, 309.
Sneddon, I. B. (1951). *Trans. Ass. ind. med. Offrs.*, 1, 142.
Sneddon, I. B., and Archibald, R. McL. (1958). *Br. J. Derm.*, 70, 211.
Teleky, L. (1948). *History of Factory and Mine Hygiene.* Columbia University Press, New York.
Thackrah, C. T. (1832). *The Effects of Arts, Trades, and Professions, and of Civic States and Habits of Living, on Health and Longevity*, 2nd ed. Longman, London.
Watkins, J. T., Hunt, T. A., Fernandez, R. H. P., and Edwards, O. P. (1958). *Br. J. ind. Med.,* 15, 105.
White, R. Prosser (1915). *Occupational Affections of the Skin*, 1st ed. H. K. Lewis, London.
White, R. Prosser (1928). *The Dermatergoses or Occupational Affections of the Skin*, 3rd ed. H. K. Lewis, London.
Willan, R. (1808). *Description and Treatment of Cutaneous Diseases*, Vol. I. *On Cutaneous Diseases.* J. Johnson, London.
Williamson, D. M., and Vickers, H. R. (1972). In *Medicine in the Mining Industries,* edited by J. M. Rogan, p. 178. Heinemann, London.
Wilson, A., and Levy, H. (1939). *Workmen's Compensation,* Vol. 1, p. 17. Oxford University Press, London.
Zackheim, H. S., and Pinkus, H. (1957) *A.M.A. Archs. Derm.*, 76, 244.

ACKNOWLEDGEMENT

I wish to thank the National Coal Board, Dr John Rogan the Chief Medical Officer and other officers of the Medical Department, for much helpful advice and permission to refer to the Annual Report 1971-72.

THE PLACE OF NICKEL IN THE HISTORY OF INDUSTRIAL DISEASE

J. GWYNNE MORGAN

Nickel and copper ore look very similar to one another and from this fact nickel came to get its name. About 200 years ago, when some miners in Saxony were mining for copper, they brought to the surface an ore which looked like copper ore. When they smelted it, a white metal was obtained which they did not recognise. Copper itself is a soft metal easy to work. This was so hard that they could not do anything with it for, in those days, if a metal was not soft enough to hammer into the shape one wanted, it was not of much use. The Saxon miners, being very superstitious and believing in spells and witchcraft, thought that Satan—or ' Old Nick '—had cast a spell over their mine, and so they named this new metal '*Kupfer-Nickel*', or ' Old Nick's Copper '.

In 1751 Alex Cronstedt (1) described to the Swedish Academy of Science his discovery of a new metal resembling *Kupfer-Nickel* which he had isolated from an ore containing iron, cobalt and copper. He dropped the '*Kupfer*' and called the new metal ' Nickel '.

Nickel had already been used in the Far East, where the Chinese had been making ornaments from a white metal called *paitung*, made by adding zinc to nickel. When trade routes were opened with China in the seventeenth century the East India Company brought back to Germany articles made of *paitung*. Soon vases and decorative pieces were being made in Europe from a metal alloy of zinc and nickel, called German silver. In 1881 the first nickel coins were issued in Switzerland.

The greatest impetus to the use of nickel was given when James Riley (2) presented to the British Iron and Steel Institute an historic paper which demonstrated that nickel conferred on steel qualities of toughness and strength hitherto unknown—qualities whose importance was quickly realized by the makers and users of armour plate—one of the principal markets for high quality steel at that time.

Most of the ore came from Norway and French New Caledonia but in 1883, in the course of constructing the Canadian Pacific Railroad, a rich outcrop of ore was discovered near Sudbury, Ontario, Canada. This appeared to be copper ore but the first batch was found to be contaminated by a large quantity of nickel.

The centre of metallurgy at this time was in and around Swansea under the direction of the Vivian family who, quick to realize the importance of nickel, bought some land near Sudbury, where they built the Victoria Mine. The ore was imported to Swansea to be treated at Messrs Vivian's works at Upper Bank, by an expensive wet process but which yielded only 40% pure nickel.

A young chemist named Langer, working on the use of nickel for batteries at a laboratory run by the Mond family at Petit France, London inadvertently spilt a solution of nickel salts on to his Bunsen gas burner. Later he noticed nickel had been deposited on the burner itself, and on investigation, found that the nickel from the salts had combined with the carbon monoxide to form nickel carbonyl (the nickel carbonyl being decomposed by the hot stem of the Bunsen burner to deposit pure nickel on it). In 1890 Langer and Quincke (3) reported this in a paper at the Institute of Chemistry. Dr Ludwig Mond (father of Sir Alfred Mond) quickly realizing the importance of the discovery set Langer to make practical use of it.

A pilot plant was built at Birmingham in 1898 and by 1900 Langer was ready to produce a refining plant. A site for this plant was needed which had available port facilities for the delivery of ore from Canada, coal and water. A location fulfilling all these conditions was found at Clydach, near Swansea.

The ore contained nickel, copper, iron and small amounts of precious metals. The iron and silica were removed leaving a nickel matte, from which the nickel was extractable either by an electrolytic process in Canada or by a carbonyl process at Clydach.

At Clydach the matte was crushed and ground to a fine powder, then heated in calciners to form oxides of nickel before reduction by water gas at a temperature of 300—350°C. The reduced matte was fed into volatilisers where carbon monoxide was passed over it and the nickel converted into nickel carbonyl. The gaseous nickel carbonyl was introduced into decomposers where it passed over nickel pellets heated to 180°C, becoming dissociated and depositing pure nickel on the heated pellets. Many modifications in the process have been made including the introduction of modern methods of dust suppression at every stage. The erection of the plant at Clydach commenced in 1900 and was commissioned in 1902. The nickel produced at Clydach was 99.99% pure and produced at a very low cost.

The ore from Canada also contained precious metals such as gold, platinum, rhodium, ruthenium. These were separated from the nickel at Clydach and sent to a precious metals refinery, specially built at Acton. The copper in the ore was produced as copper sulphate, which was mostly sent to France for spraying on the vines.

Dr Langer was a man of great vision who not only planned the works at Clydach on the most modern lines, but had great ideas in regard to welfare. Houses were built for the workmen and the Mond Institute for their recreation which contained a concert hall, billiard hall, library and photographic facilities. In addition he encouraged the formation of a brass band, a football team, and other sporting facilities. He was also one of the first employers to commence a pension scheme.

Dr Langer soon realized that he was dealing with a highly toxic substance and so all precautions were taken in the design of the plant for safeguarding the operatives. Despite this, however, some cases of nickel carbonyl poisoning did occur in the first few months of the operation of the new plant at Clydach. Research into the toxic properties of the new compound was accordingly undertaken by A. Mosso and Armit (4), Tunicliffe (6), Professor Haldane (5), and Sir John Rose Bradford. They suggested that a level of 0.5% of nickel carbonyl was dangerous, but later investigations have shown that even this level was far too high. In fact the threshold limit value as suggested by the American Conference of Governmental Industrial Hygienists is 0.001 parts per million.

The symptoms of acute poisoning may be immediate or delayed. Often they are ushered in by retrosternal pain following the initial symptoms of dizziness, headache, and nausea. These merge gradually into the delayed reaction in about ten to fourteen hours, with its attack of coughing and dyspnoea.

During World War One, the Germans first used chlorine as a poisonous gas. The symptoms were well known and thus the gravity of each case could be assessed. The Germans later used phosgene which is really a carbonyl, being produced by the action of carbon monoxide upon chlorine. The patient admitted to a first aid post, apparently soon recovered and was sent back to the trenches only to succumb to the delayed reaction. The poisonous effect of the carbonyls is on the respiratory system, where it lowers the oxygenating capacity of the blood.

Various chemical methods have been attempted to remove nickel from the body and substances known as chelating agents have proved successful. Barnes and Denz (7) of the British Research Council investigated the use of British Anti-Lewisite on rabbits poisoned by nickel carbonyl, and found that the mortality rates were greatly reduced. Acting on the fact that EDTA (a salt of ethylene diamine tetra-acetic acid) has a chelating effect on lead, it was found that it also had a chelating effect on nickel (J. Gwynne Morgan). The acute symptoms subsided in a shorter time than in former cases. There was also an increase of nickel excreted in the urine. This then became the standard form of treatment. EDTA was superseded by a more efficient chelating agent known as dithiocarbamate. Sunderman (8) reported excellent results by the use of dithiocarbamate on eleven persons after exposure to nickel carbonyl in a factory in the U.S.A.

For the formation of nickel carbonyl, large amounts of carbon monoxide are used and there are occasional leaks giving rise to carbon monoxide poisoning. Another industrial hazard found to be associated with the production of nickel was that of nickel dermatitis. Sensitivity to nickel was first described by Lain (9) who observed three cases of dermatitis due to nickel plated spectacle frames. From medical examination of new entrants to the Clydach works by means of the patch test, it was found that 3% were allergic to nickel, a figure which agrees with that of other investigators on its incidence amongst the general public. Ancillary to the process of refining nickel, nickel salts were also produced. It was amongst those working with these salts that nickel dermatitis occurred. Bulmer & McKenzie (10) found that nickel rashes occurred in those people with high alkaline sweat and advised administration of calcium chloride which counteracts the tendency towards alkalosis.

Nickel is usually regarded as one of the non-toxic metals in comparison with lead, copper and mercury. Extensive investigations carried out in foreign countries, notably in Austria, Russia and the United States, appeared to show that no danger was likely to arise from the use of nickel cooking vessels. After the sudden illness of the Emperor of Austria, blame was attributed to the use in the royal kitchen of new cooking utensils made from nickel. A law was passed in 1887 (11) forbidding the use of nickel in the manufacture of cooking utensils. However, Roos (12) after feeding his family for a year on food cooked in nickel utensils was able to prove at the sixth International Congress that the cooking of food in nickel utensils was not detrimental to health and the Congress passed a resolution to this effect. This evidence was passed to the Austrian authorities who repealed the Act (13).

It was noticed that after the nickel refining process had been in operation for about thirty years, several deaths from respiratory cancer occurred. The first account of lung cancer associated with nickel refining was published in the Report of the Eighth International Congress for Occupational diseases by Amor (14). Professor Bradford Hill (15) was approached with a view to obtaining statistical information as to its significance. He found that not only was there an apparent and abnormal incidence of carcinoma of the lung and nose in the refinery population from 1929 to 1938, but that the excess was confined to the process workers.

Men who had entered the Clydach works after a certain period were not affected, and so a register of all entrants was prepared to delineate separately the cause and year of death. It became apparent that the highest incidence of cancer of the lung and nose occurred in those workers who began work between 1905 and 1914. Thereafter there was a progressive fall until 1920, when the incidence rose again. This was, however, of short duration. It is of great significance that no nasal cases were recorded in any person who entered the works for the first time after 1924; and only six lung cases had occurred, which figure is well within the number of cases expected from the country rate (Morgan [16]).

In 1958, Doll (17) found that the number of deaths observed from lung cancer amongst nickel workers engaged before 1924 was nearly five times the expected rate, but this risk has been largely removed in the last 35 years.

As an index of the action of any carcinogenic material which had been present in the nickel works, the incidence of nasal cancer was far more significant than that of lung cancer. A study of the occupational histories revealed that the hazard related to those engaged in dusty occupations such as calcination, manufacture of copper sulphate and the furnaces, and there was a long time lapse between the exposure to risk and the onset of cancer. This lag period is enhanced by several factors such as age at entry into the occupation, length of service, individual susceptibility and the concentration of the carcinogen. It is interesting that the lag period is similar to that of bladder cancer in the rubber industry, lung cancer in the workers in the Schneeburg mines and workers in the chrome industry.

The pertinent questions were why did the cases cease in men engaged after 1924 and what had been the carcionogen ? There was a difficulty in that several things happened in 1924, namely :

(1) A more efficient type of calciner was installed.
(2) Sulphuric acid containing arsenic was replaced with arsenic-free sulphuric acid.
(3) The copper sulphate plant was closed (thus again eliminating sulphuric acid).
(4) A Lodge Cottrell electrostatic precipitator was installed which diminished the amount of dust in the plant.
(5) Dust-proof respirators were worn by all process men.

It seemed likely that it was therefore the heated dust which contained the carcinogen. Before 1924 this dust contained arsenic from the sulphuric acid used.

My enquiries have covered over fifty years of industrial data. They involved an exhaustive study of all available information about persons who had worked in the industry and were known to have suffered from the diseases described above. During the period of decades it may take to arrive at a substantive solution to a problem on medical research, perspectives are apt to be both biased and clouded, often hampered by high hopes and by unsubstantiated sensational claims. Nevertheless an appraisal of many solid facts and the present trend towards study of mechanisms leads to the conclusion that this field will contribute to a better comprehension of the cancer problem.

REFERENCES

1 Cronstedt, A. F. (1751). Förfök giorde med en malmart frän Los kobolt grufvor Färila socken och Helsingeland. *K. sevenska VetenskAkad. Handl.*, 12, 287.

2 Riley, J. (1889). Alloys of nickel and steel. *J. Iron Steel Inst.*, p. 45.

3 Mond, L., Langer, C., and Quincke, F. (1890). Action of carbon monoxide on nickel. *J. chem. Soc.*, 57, 749.

4 Armit, H. W. (1907). The toxicology of nickel carbonyl. I. *J. Hyg.*, 7, 525. —(1908). The Toxicology of nickel carbonyl. II. *J. Hyg.*, 8, 565.

5 Haldane, . (1895). The action of carbonic oxide on man. *J. Physiol.*, 18, 430.

6 Tunnicliffe, F. W., and Plimmer, H. G. (1903). Report to Mond Nickel Company of results of a post-mortem : a fatal case at Clydach.

7 Barnes, J. M., and Denz, F. A. (1951). The effect of 2-3 dimercapto-propanol (B.A.L.) on experimental nickel carbonyl poisoning. *Br. J. ind. Med.*, 8, 117.

8 Sunderman, F. W., Sr., and Sunderman, F. W., Jr. (1958). Nickel poisoning. VIII. Dithiocarb : a new therapeutic agent for persons exposed to nickel carbonyl. *Am. J. med. Sci.*, 236, 26.

9 Lain, E. S. (1931). Nickel dermatitis : a new source. *J. Am. med. Ass.*, 96, 771-772.

10 Bulmer, F.M.R., and McKenzie, E. A. (1947). *Canad. chem. Process. Ind.*, 31, 524, 525.

11 Austrian Law (1884). Decree passed forbidding use of nickel for cooking utensils.

12 Van Roos (1887). *6th int. Congr. Hyg., Vienna.*

13 Austrian Law (1897). Repeal of 1884 Law.

14 Amor, A. J. (1939). Resumé of growths of respiratory tract which occurred in a nickel refinery. *Rep. 8th int. Congr. ind. Accid. occup. Dis., Leipzig*, 1938, 2, 941.

15 Hill, A. B. (1939). Report to Mond Nickel Company.

16 Morgan, J. G. (1958). Some observations on the incidence of respiratory cancer in nickel workers. *Brit. J. ind. Med.*, 15, 224.

17 Doll, R. (1958). Cancer of the lung and nose in nickel workers. *Br. J. ind. Med.*, 15, 217.

THE HISTORY OF BRUCELLOSIS IN WALES

EIRIAN WILLIAMS

None so blind as those that will not see.
None so deaf as those that will not hear.

There are three main species in the genus *brucella, br. abortus, br. melitensis* and *br. suis* and their definitive hosts are the cow, the goat and the pig. Luckily in Wales as in the rest of Britain *br. abortus* is the only enzootic species, for the illness in man is usually less severe than *melitensis or suis brucellosis* and is rarely fatal. It is primarily an occupational disease, the result of contact with infected animals or contaminated implements, and farm workers, slaughtermen, veterinary surgeons and agricultural engineers are mostly at risk. Others, foolishly or unknowingly, drink raw milk.

Brucellosis by repute is a disease of antiquity but its early history is uncertain and is a fertile field for sterile conjecture. Jacob appealed to Laban the Syrian when pursued into the mountains of Gilead 'This twenty years have I been with thee : thy ewes and thy she goats have not cast their young'. And there are references also to large scale epizootics in and beyond the early Christian era. Abortion or premature labour, however, has many causes—salmonellosis, for example, is fast becoming pre-eminent, and brucellosis cannot be blamed for all outbreaks of bovine contagious abortion in Wales in years gone by. It was recognised in Britain more than 400 years ago and Mascall, in 1587, spoke of 'divers approved remedies to helpe most diseases among cattell', abortion included.[1] It could be argued that the direction of spread was from England into Wales, as it may have been to America in the wake of the Pilgrim Fathers, for according to Barlow, in 1851, cattle in the mountainous districts of Wales and Scotland were spared when disease had already become established in the richer districts of the Kingdom.[2]

By the nineteenth century contagious abortion was known to be a serious enervating burden on our livestock industry. In 1816, a veterinary surgeon, John Edwards, of the Vale of Clwyd, warned that it resulted in serious loss, that cows in prime condition were especially vulnerable, and that the foul emanation from carcasses rotting in grass or lightly covered with soil was responsible.[3] Modern farmers would proclaim John Edwards a true prophet of doom, knowing to their cost that *br. abortus* thrives in lush pasture and that abortion storms may ensue when diseased herds are replaced prematurely. Bernhard Bang, a Danish physician turned veterinary pathologist, first identified *br. abortus* on December 19, 1895, in uterine exudate from a cow showing signs of impending abortion but in Wales routine diagnostic facilities were not available until Veterinary Investigation Centres were established, firstly in Cardiff in 1922 and later in Bangor, Aberystwyth and Carmarthen.[4] In Bangor, in 1931 and 1932, 16.5% of the cows in 52 milking herds were shown to be infected, although in a national survey in 1964, the lowest herd incidence was in Wales—12%, and the highest in neighbouring English counties—almost 30%.[5] Some of the changes in the regional and local incidence of brucellosis can be explained. Before the turn of the century traffic was outward from Wales—black Castle Martins and other Welsh runts for fattening and slaughter—trekking along ancient drovers' routes, our traditional highways for commerce, banditry and adventure. With the change to milk production the trend was reversed and Friesian and other better milking breeds were introduced, mostly from England, bringing with them new invigorating admixtures of brucella strains. Thus, in 1968, when farms in Cheshire and north Wales were re-stocked after foot and mouth disease, infection was often due to *br. abortus* biotype 5, a strain hitherto usually encountered in Scotland and in the north of England.[6] 'Flying herds' whose unproductive cows are ruthlessly replaced to maintain a high milk yield, understandably, are often heavily infected. A strict rule on some small farms however is never to introduce new stock. Animals are all home reared. But even in this seemingly safe environment brucellosis can suddenly take its toll and then the fox is blamed, or any other scavenger happening by. Foxes travel far, and some, tagged as cubs, have been caught eight miles from home. In a recent survey involving eighty-seven foxes in west Wales eight gave positive results when blood was tested for brucella antibodies. In one, *br. abortus* type 1 was identified, proving for the first time that the British red fox can become infected.[7] There is no evidence however that he also transmits the disease.

Man, earth's busiest migrant, denied his role as a vector of bovine pathogens until *Salmonella dublin* was isolated from pustules on the arms of a veterinary surgeon, examined while still at work.[8,9,10.] He was one of fifty-seven in a series of sixty-two in Wales who performed obstetric procedures without wearing gloves. More than a century ago the ill-fated Ignaz Philipp Semmelweis, of the Allgemeines Krankenhaus, Vienna, showed that puerperal fever in women was spread by doctors and students commuting, unwashed, from post-mortems to lying-in wards. But it does not follow that veterinary surgeons who do not practise strict asepsis are the main vectors of brucellosis, salmonellosis and other contagions in cows. While infection in the parturient woman is established by inserting streptococci in the genital tract, and, experimentally, Bernhard Bang also infected cows *per vaginam*, in nature brucellosis is not carried in this way.[11] Its mode of entry on the farms of Wales, therefore, cannot always be explained and the stealth and unpredictability of its treacherous visitations remain a mystery and a challenge.

PIONEERS OF BRUCELLA RESEARCH AND THEIR WELSH CONNECTION

Surgeon Captain Matthew Louis Hughes

Marston may have been the first to describe brucellosis in man but Louis Hughes in his classic monograph *Mediterranean, Malta, or Undulant Fever* gave the earliest authoritative account of the disease.[12] It was based on his experience as a surgeon captain in the Army serving in Malta and is still unsurpassed as a reference book for clinicians. He coined the name ' Undulant fever ' and also the epithet ' Melitensis ' which has been retained for the caprine species. At the age of thirty-two, two years after his work was published, he died ministering to the wounded, one of many casualties in an ill-conceived attack on a Boer position outside Ladysmith.[13] According to Sir Patrick Manson it was ' the untimely death of an ideal Army Surgeon, soldierly in his bearing and gentle as a physician ever should be '.

His greatgrandfather, Edward Hughes, baptized in Whitford, Flintshire, had moved to London in 1758 but ties of a kind with Wales must have been retained for in the preface to the *Conway Parish Register* of 1900, is the entry ' There is only one whom this message cannot reach—Captain Matthew Louis Hughes, R.A.M.C., killed at the battle of Colenso, December 15, 1899 '.[14] With others who died in the Boer War, he may also have been commemorated on a monument near Cardiff's City Hall, but names facing west, beneath the heading ' Army Medical Service ', have faded and in our capital, regrettably, now there is no official record.

In Malta, Louis Hughes met and married Kate Winifred, the daughter of Dr Henry Simpson, of Colwyn Bay and of Bowden in Cheshire. Both contracted Malta Fever in 1896.

Miss Alice C. Evans (1881-)

Surgeon Major David Bruce had reported his finding of a micrococcus, the cause of Malta Fever, in 1887, and in 1895 Professor Bernhard Bang had described the bacillus of bovine contagious abortion. Their choice of generic names *micrococcus* and *bacillus* was unfortunate. It meant that the recognition of the near kinship of these two organisms was delayed, knowledge about brucellosis in its many guises remained scant and confused and the suggestion that human disease might be caused by bacillus abortus was rejected. In 1917 Alice Evans, a bacteriologist in the United States Department of Agriculture in Washington, was studying the bacterial flora of fresh milk.[15] She was inspired to compare Bruce's *micrococcus melitensis* with Bang's *bacillus* and, as she later explained, it was the fact that both organisms were known to be excreted in the milk of apparently healthy animals suggested this comparison. To her confessed amazement they were identical in morphology, biochemical reactions and in their reactions in abortus antiserum—a discovery of outstanding importance. She postulated ' The very close relationship between Bact. abortus and an organism pathogenic to human beings adds a new interest to the question of the possible pathogenicity of Bact. abortus to human subjects '—in its time an observation of equally outstanding impertinence. But proof came in 1924 when Orpen in South Africa isolated *br. abortus* from patients who had been in contact only with infected cows. This work by Alice Evans was greeted at first with universal scepticism but is now acclaimed. Her contributions were not only in bacteriology. She also wrote ably on clinical diagnosis, emphasizing from experience as a patient the danger of confusing organic with psychoneurotic disease. Her symptoms had been due to brucellosis but doctors were determinedly unconvinced until brucella organisms were isolated from lesions found at laparotomy—a humbling, cautionary tale for all who profess to practise medicine. She became Senior Bacteriologist to the National Institute of Health in Washington where she remained until retirement in 1945. Her home now is in Alexandria, Virginia. In September, 1973, she described how her paternal grandparents had emigrated to Pennsylvania in 1831 from Clyneithrim Farm, Llangyfelach Parish, near Pontardawe.[16] Her mother, Anne B. Evans, left Rhysurdareth, near Newport, Monmouthshire in 1861. She herself was born in Neath, Pennsylvania, an exclusively Welsh rural community.

DISCOVERING HUMAN BR. ABORTUS INFECTION IN WALES AND ELSEWHERE

In 1914, Major J. C. Kennedy, a member of the Mediterranean Fever Commission wrote 'In placing on record the fact that in high dilutions the milk and the blood serum of certain cows in London dairies agglutinate the micrococcus melitensis I do not wish to appear an alarmist. I do not wish to be understood to say that the cows are therefore capable of transmitting undulant fever. It is possible that this agglutination reaction of the milk may have some explanation other than that the cows are infected with the micrococcus melitensis . . .'[17] The true explanation, by Alice Evans, that melitensis antibodies were produced in response to abortus infection was at first rejected and probably because the world was then at war the controversy received little attention. Gradually it became clear that *br. abortus*, as well as *br. melitensis*, was harmful to man and case reports appeared in evidence. In Britain, Dr Theodore Thompson, Physician to the London Hospital, is credited with the seventh.[18] On June 1, 1928, his patient, a gentleman farmer and a native of Cumberland, had felt seedy and had shivered. The following day he was able to motor 300 miles to attend a regimental dinner but on June 13th he had three rigors. He remained unwell and had more rigors until the third week. Leucopenia was noted and his blood was found to contain brucella antibodies. It was then discovered that four cows and two heifers on his farm had recently aborted. A comprehensive review of the literature accompanied this lucid report, and Dr William Evans, First Assistant, was thanked for preparing notes. Its style and construction seemed familiar and in the pursuit of historical exactitude Dr Evans, once more of Tregaron, which is in the middle of Cardiganshire, was asked, and he replied, 'Yes, I wrote the paper, and paid for the typing '.[19]

HUMAN BRUCELLOSIS REPORTED IN WALES

Brucellosis was diagnosed for the first time in Wales at the Cardiff Royal Infirmary.[20] Late in July, 1928, a director of music had toured the Highlands of Scotland, consuming raw milk and cream on the way. Early in October he became feverish with sweats of moderate severity. They became profuse, often drenching, with a peculiar and disagreeable odour and recurring almost daily until December 21st, when a small foul smelling part of necrosed bone was extruded into the mouth. The patient's serum on November 23rd contained antibodies to *br. abortus* in a dilution of 1 in 250 and on March 20th, 1929, in a dilution of 1 in 1000. This was also the first described example of brucella osteomyelitis involving the jaw.

HUMAN BRUCELLOSIS ACQUIRED IN WALES

Dr Roland Williams of Maenclochog

It was Dr Roland Williams of Maenclochog, Pembrokeshire, who first diagnosed brucellosis acquired from a native cow.[21] In January, 1930, he visited a farmer, aged 53, who appeared to be suffering from influenza but his spleen became palpable and his blood was then found to contain antibodies to *brucella abortus* in high dilution. Veterinary surgeons confirmed that epidemic abortion was especially rife among cattle in the village, and the farmer said that four of his cows had lost their calves in the preceding six months. One had aborted three weeks before he had first complained of symptoms and into this cow he had inserted pessaries manually to ' help clear her up '. The farm, several miles downhill towards the Landsker from Maenclochog, under new ownership, is now brucella free. It has an important place in history but to forestall unwanted notoriety it will not be named.

Roland Williams was a clinician of wide experience and repute and also a keen antiquarian.[22] In the History of Medicine Section of the Annual Meeting of the British Medical Association held in Cardiff in 1928 he read a paper entitled ' Welsh Physicians and the Renaissance ' and is remembered more recently for the tours he led through the mountains, retracing the forgotten byways of our heritage.[23] Maenclochog, nestled under Moelcwmcerwyn on the brow of Mynydd Presely is within walking distance of Cerrig y Marchogion, Carn Meini and Carn Alw whence came the blue stones of Stone Henge. Aloft clings a prehistoric track trampled in latter days by furtively driven Irish cattle, bringing their own heady brucella brew. There are signs of a Roman way and at remote Carnabwth once lived Twm Becca, leader of the rebellious Daughters of Rebecca who, disguised as women, wrecked turnpikes and tollgates to the delight of the drovers and to the relief of the poor—' And they blessed Rebekah and said unto her, be thou the mother of thousands of ten thousands and let thy seed possess the gate of those which hate them '.

Roland Williams died on April 14, 1968, and in Maenclochog churchyard a simple Presely stone marks his grave. He was born in 1891 in Llanbedr, Merionethshire. His father, the Rev. George Williams, once a shepherd boy in Llanuwchllyn, was Minister of Ainon, Church of the Particular Baptists in Harlech and also of Salem, the famous old chapel in Cefncymmerau. Salem is now immortalized in Vosper's depiction of our traditional puritanical way of life.

THE DELAY IN DISCOVERING BRUCELLOSIS IN WALES

Common transmitted diseases, among them typhoid, diphtheria and tuberculosis, were described long before bacteria were classified. In Wales brucellosis was a notable exception and the delay until 1929, now, with hindsight, might seem inexplicable. Its symptoms however were non-specific ; there was no exanthem or any other distinctive sign and unlike the disease in Malta, brucellosis in Wales was rarely fatal. That life for our people early this century was precarious is starkly conveyed in the first report of Pembrokeshire's Medical Officer of Health. It also shows brucellosis in perspective. In 1911 the population of the county was 89,850. One hundred and fifty-four cases of diphtheria were reported and twenty-three died. There were nine deaths from typhoid, one hundred and one from phthisis, twenty-three from tuberculous meningitis and thirty from tuberculosis presenting in other ways. The County Medical Officer of Health, Dr H. O. Williams, estimated that there were 400 patients in Pembrokeshire suffering from pulmonary tuberculosis and that a quarter would die within the year. Most of them lived in damp dark overcrowded cottages with no hope of recovery. While the death rate from phthisis in males was below the national average, in females it was very much higher for '. . . the women never get fresh air. After breathing foul air throughout the night they have to work in it all day. They never get out except on Sundays when they go from a stuffy house into an equally stuffy church or chapel '. Brucellosis, recognised, would have been stoically received.

THE DELAY IN ERADICATION

The deadlier contagions have been contained and today we revere an aging welfare state. Brucellosis is witness to its frailty and imperfection. Elsewhere the disease has disappeared but in Wales it thrives because eradication has been judged on financial grounds regardless of human risk.[24] (Table 1) And significantly those most at risk, farm workers and smallholders, if not inarticulate are the least complaining. An excuse has been that the incidence of human brucellosis is unknown but reports have reliably confirmed that it is an inevitable hazard where bovine disease is rife.[25,26,27,28] The illness varies in severity. It can be mild, allowing work—though many patients stay at work because they have no alternative—or disabling and protracted. Some are discovered only after enquiry, relatives, for example, of known patients or cowmen attached to 'flying herds', a notoriously dangerous trade, and there is, therefore, no reliable index of occupational morbidity. In 1957 Davies described eleven patients with brucellosis from one rural practice in Carmarthen and now in south-west Wales some thirty patients are diagnosed each year.[29]

Table 1

Campaigns for the Eradication of Bovine Brucellosis.
Modified from Stableforth 1969[24]

	Position before Campaign	*Latest position known*
Norway	1936 27.9% herds free	1953 All herds free
Sweden	1938 5.5% herds infected	1958 All herds free
Finland	1939 3443 herds infected	1960 All herds free
Denmark	1946 25% herds infected	1962 All herds free
German Fed. Rep.	1956 5% herds infected	1964 All herds free
Netherlands	1954 30% herds infected	1968 99.95% herds free
Austrian Rep.	1958 4.7% infected animals	1968 99.58% herds free
Northern Ireland	1960 About 15% herds infected	1969 98.3% herds free

Table 2

BRUCELLOSIS ACQUIRED FROM MILK

BRUCELLOSIS IN SOUTH WEST WALES
(Not Including Veterinary Surgeons)
100 *Consecutive Patients Presenting Until Early* 1972

OCCUPATIONAL 85%		NON-OCCUPATIONAL 15% (From Infected Milk)	
Farmers or farm workers	68	Housewives	6
Farmers' wives	6	Students	2
Farmers' sons	4	Army major	1
Slaughtermen	4	Hospital lab. technician	1
Milk lorry driver	1	Hospital nurse	1
Agricultural engineer	1	Forestry mechanic	1
Daughter of agricultural engineer	1	Teacher	1
		Builder	1
		Bank Clerk	1

Attitudes in Wales to milk are pre-Listerian and students at university trustingly drink it raw.[30] Reading the story of brucellosis, however, from the time it was first recognised, on for thirty years, the wary will wonder at the Milk and Dairies (General) Regulations 1959.[31] This document and a later circular give guidance to local authorities concerning the sale of raw milk—ineffectual guidance.[32] Their real achievement is to give licence to producer retailers of raw infected milk. Local authorities are discouraged from withdrawing retailing licences unless *br. abortus* can be isolated from it.[33] Some authorities do not bother to try. Others do but have found this to be uncertain evidence of bovine infection. Reprehensibly, for many years one branch of government has had proof of infection in herds because of proper tests in veterinary laboratories, while another branch of government has condoned the sale of raw milk from the same herds. The first branch is the Ministry of Agriculture, Fisheries and Food, and the Department of Health is the second—and its prolongation this way to The Welsh Office is not without blame.

The collusion involving Government, certain local authorities and a few farmers, to persuade the innocent to drink infected milk will make sorry history. A forestry mechanic with acute brucellosis had raw infected milk delivered to his door.[34] It came from the farm of a licensed producer retailer. The Ministry of Agriculture, Fisheries and

Food knew the milk was infected but the licensing authority did not because its own tests had been perfunctory and negative. The Ministry had not warned the licensing authority that the cows' milk was infected because it wished to retain the confidence of farmers. So much for the milk of human kindness.

A nurse was supplied with raw infected milk by a licensed producer retailer, whose head cowman had presented with brucellosis a year before. The local authority had then been asked to place a pasteurization order but had refused. When the nurse became ill the authority was again asked and again refused. The farmer was visited and was asked not to sell raw milk, but he refused. Practising veterinary surgeons knew this herd was infected, the Ministry of Agriculture knew the herd was infected.[33] Indeed almost every department of Government should have known it was infected except perhaps the Foreign Office and no action was ever taken. Thus is the making of sorry history.

CONCLUSION

Eradication at long last has started. But it will take time. Proudly, Wales will then have joined the ranks of the developed nations.

REFERENCES

1 Mascall, L. *The first booke of Cattell*, J. Wolfe, London, 1587.
2 Barlow, J. *Jl R. agric. Soc.* (1851), 12, 62.
3 Edwards, J. *Y Cyfarwyddyd Profedig i Bob Perchen Anifeiliaid* . . . T. Gee, Denbigh, 1816.
4 Williams, B. M. Personal Communication.
5 Animal Disease Surveys. Report No. 4 : *Brucellosis in the British Dairy Herd*, by F. B. Leech, *et al.* H. M. S. Office, London, 1964.
6 Rowland, W. T. Personal Communication.
7 Davies, G. Personal Communication.
8 Williams, E. British Veterinary Congress 1968 (Unpublished).
9 Bell, P. *Br. Fmr.* (1968) November 2nd, 28.
10 Williams, E. *Lancet* (1969), 2, 737.
11 Bang, B. *J. Comp. Path.* (1897), 10, 125.
12 Hughes, M. L. *Mediterranean, Malta or Undulant Fever.* Macmillan, London, 1897.
13 Hughes, G. W. G. and Hughes, M. H. *Jl R. Army med. Cps* (1969), 115, 198.
14 Hughes, M. H. Personal Communication.
15 Evans, A. C. *J. infect. Dis.* (1918), 22, 580.
16 Evans, A. C. Personal Communication.
17 Kennedy, J. C. *Jl R. Army med. Cps.* (1914), 22, 9.
18 Thompson, T. *Lancet* (1928), 2, 1335.
19 Evans, W. Personal Communication.
20 Davies, I. J., and Anderson W. C. *Br. med.J.* (1929), 2, 12.
21 Williams, E. R., and Sladden, A. F. *ibid.* (1930), 1, 859.
22 Williams, E. R. *North Pembrokeshire*, Great Western Railway, London 1936.
23 Williams, E. R. *Br. med. J.* (1928), 2, 1133.
24 Stableforth, A. W. *Proc. R. agric. Soc. Clth.* Report of the Fourth Conference, held in Nairobi in September, 1969. Nairobi, 1971.
25 Barrett, G. M., and Rickards, A. G. *Q. Jl Med.* (1953), 22, 23.
26 Dalrymple-Champneys, W. *Brucella Infection and Undulant Fever in Man.* Oxford University Press, London 1960.
27 Bothwell, P. W. in *Some Diseases of Animals Communicable to Man in Britain*, edited by O. Graham-Jones, Pergamon, Oxford, 1968.
28 Williams, E. *Lancet* (1970), 1, 604.
29 Davies J. E. *Br. med. J.* (1957), 4, 1082.
30 Williams, E. *ibid* (1971), 3, 45.
31 *The Milk and Dairies (General) Regulations:* 1959. H.M.S.O., London, 1959 S.I. No. 277.
32 Ministry of Health Circular 17/66.
33 Williams, E. *Lancet* (1970), 1, 1220.
34 Williams, E. *Br. med. J.* (1973), 1, 791.

SIR JOHN WILLIAMS (1840—1926)
HIS BACKGROUND AND ACHIEVEMENT*

EMYR WYN JONES

On my shoulders rests the onerous duty of offering an 'Introduction to the Exhibition of Books and Manuscripts' that has been compiled and made available for inspection by the members of this Congress. My sincere gratitude for having been given this privilege is more than counterbalanced by the sense of responsibility that the task engenders.

Although the exact title restricts me to 'Books and Manuscripts' it would be churlish of me not to interpose a warm reference to all the other exhibitions, and in particular the special display that has been prepared at the Welsh Folk Museum at St Fagans. This magnificent Folk Museum is unique in the United Kingdom, and in Europe only the Scandinavian countries have anything of a similar nature to compare with it. It is also imperative that full recognition be given to various organisations and private individuals who have generously allowed the Congress to borrow some of their treasured possessions for exhibition. I know that members will join with me in thanking all these kind people for their gracious action.

But to return to my theme of 'Books and Manuscripts', I am equally sure that you would wish me to express the sincere gratitude of the Congress as a whole to the Wellcome Institute and the National Library of Wales for their very substantial support in providing valuable material for the Exhibition. The role of the Institute in these matters has been bountifully revealed on many occasions in the past, and everyone interested in medical history owes an enormous debt to the Institute.

If I appear, at this stage, to emphasise the special contribution of the National Library of Wales to the Exhibition, I trust that I shall be forgiven; because in the absence of help from the National Library

* Initial title 'Introduction to the Exhibition of Books and Manuscripts'.

there would have been available for you only a truncated and inadequate demonstration of the medical literature appertaining to Wales. It is a pleasure, therefore, to record the enthusiastic guidance that was offered to us by Mr David Jenkins, the Librarian, and his two senior officers, Mr B. G. Owens and Dr I. Moelwyn Williams. They received Dr John Cule and myself in a most friendly fashion, and gave us generously of their time and their expert knowledge of the resources of the Library. For obvious reasons some of the priceless treasures cannot be removed from the safety of the Library, but I am glad to say much rare and valuable material has been released. Furthermore, the sheer bulk of the material available compelled us to undertake a careful sifting.

It appears singularly appropriate for me to digress for a time from my main theme so as to tell the Congress something of the history of the National Library—all the more so as the story has a direct link with Swansea and its hinterland, and with the medical profession. In the early 1850's a young teenage country lad arrived in Swansea, almost certainly mounted on a Welsh Cob, to continue his education at the Normal College under the supervision of Mr Evan Davies. He had already attended the village school at Gwynfe, a remote hamlet in the hills of Carmarthenshire, and had also received further teaching at a bigger local school run by the Reverend D. Davies at Bethlehem, before venturing to Swansea. This boy, John, was the third son of David Williams, Blaenllynant, and his wife Eleanor. The father, as frequently occurred in those days, combined farming with his duties as a Congregational minister, and he was in charge of two chapels—Bethlehem, Llangadog, and Carmel, Llansadwrn,—from 1838 until 1842. As a result of his pastoral responsibilities the routine management of the farm devolved upon his wife, who must have been a remarkable woman and whose enthusiasm for hard work and education must have provided the inspiration that set her son's feet on the scholastic ladder that eventually led to the highest professional distinction.

The influence of a good mother lies behind the success story of many great men, but the maternal contribution is often incompletely recognised and inadequately recorded. Fortunately there exists a very rare booklet which gives a fascinating though brief account of the life of this particular mother, and I have not seen any reference to it elsewhere. It is written in Welsh and bears the title *Byr-gofiant am Mrs. Eleanor Williams, Talardd, Llandilo (Blaenllynant gynt)* ; it was printed by Bernard Rees a'i Fab, Argraffwyr, Llanelli, 1898. It is a small booklet of twenty pages, 7 inches by 5½ inches in size, elegantly produced and bound ; the format suggests that her (by then) very distinguished son, John, had had it published privately, and the author was her youngest son, Nathaniel, who was farming 'Glandules in the Tywi Valley'. This '*Brief Biography of Eleanor Williams*' reveals many facets of her early life and gives interesting details of the activities of the family as a whole.

Eleanor was the eldest of the twelve children of David Jones, farmer and 'freeholder' of Beili, Gwynfe, whose father had farmed Parc, between Defynnog and Brecon before coming to Beili. David Jones possessed a powerful personality and an enthusiasm for education. His wife came from the highly esteemed Lewis family of Panthowell and Pencrug, Llanddeusant. Eleanor, who was born on 29th September, 1807, had the advantage of attending a small local school at Gwynfe.

At that time the average rural school teachers were inadequate in many ways ; they have been described often enough—and many of them were discharged soldiers who had lost a limb, harboured a tempestuous temperament and were addicted to alcohol. They had had no formal training as teachers. They usually enforced discipline through fear and repression, and their threats were readily reinforced by severe corporal punishment. These methods of maintaining discipline and securing the co-operation of the children were no more prevalent in the country schools of Wales in those days than in the famous schools of England, as revealed by contemporary records, even though their headmasters might well be highly respected scholars and in Holy Orders. *O tempora* ! *O mores* !

Fortunately John Davies of Glanclydach, Eleanor's first teacher, was not in this mould. He had received a good education to prepare himself for the Ministry, and later became a farmer, and was described as an excellent schoolmaster. Later on she attended another school near Glantywi, in the Bethlehem area ; and at the age of twelve she had another year's schooling at Merthyr Tudful. Bearing in mind the dates and the general circumstances, it is evident that as a child Eleanor had had quite exceptional educational opportunities for a girl.

After returning home she worked hard on her father's farm for many years, and during this time she was a voracious reader—'read every book within reach, often until the small hourse of the morning.'

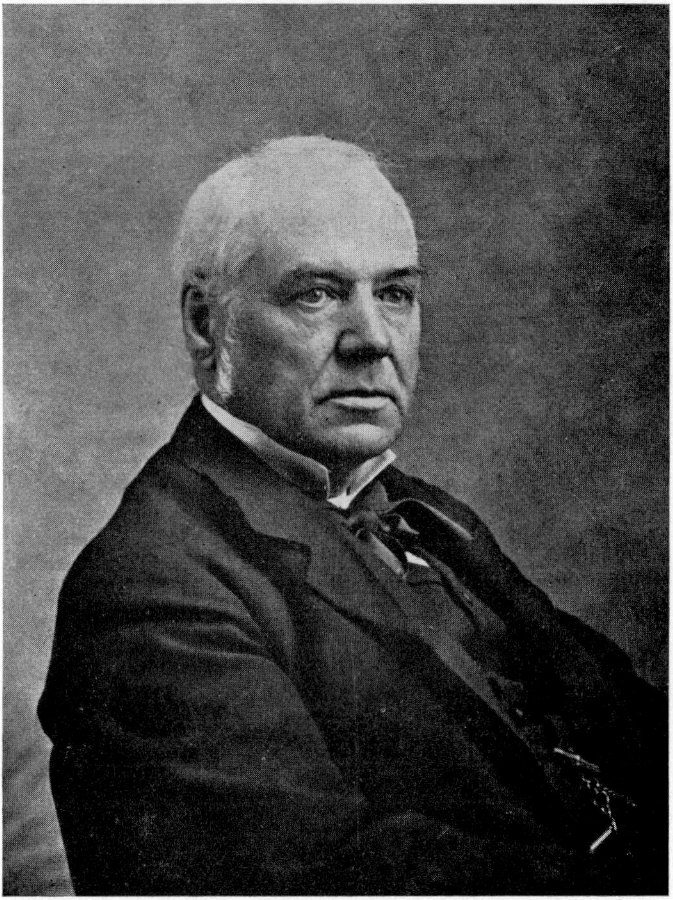

Plate 10
Sir John Williams

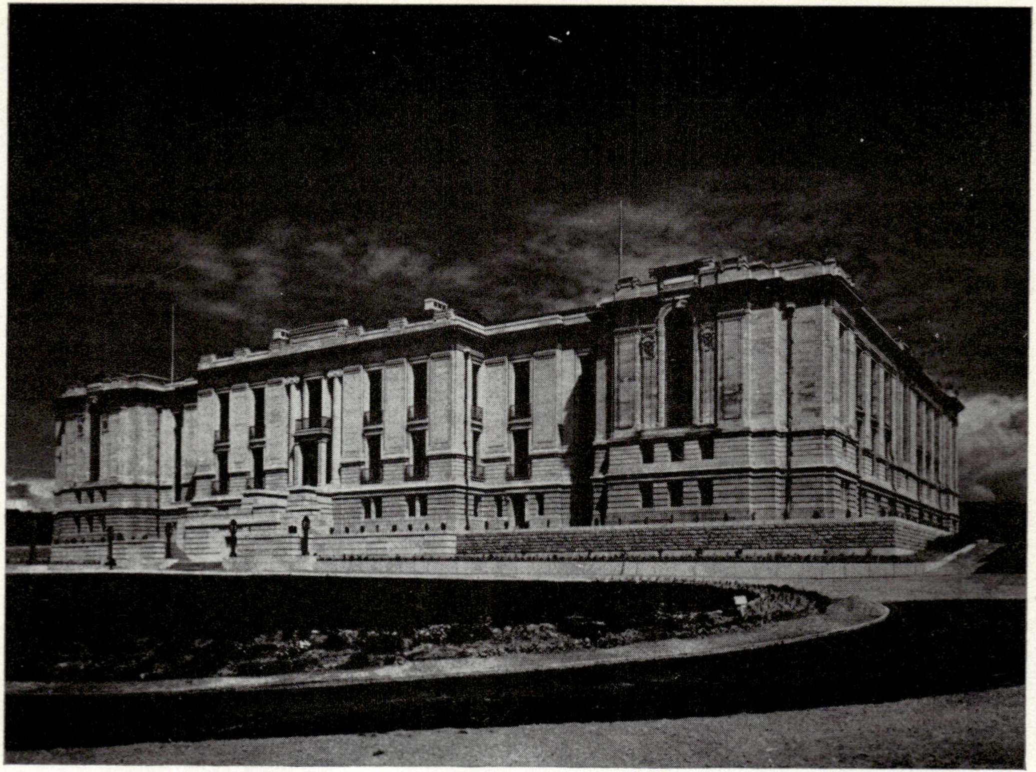

Plate II
National Library of Wales Aberystwyth

In February, 1833, she married a local man, David Williams, and joined him at his farm, Blaenllynant. In September, 1842, there was an outbreak of typhoid in the district and her husband died, leaving Eleanor to care for her sons, David, Morgan and John, and Nathaniel who was born posthumously; and to manage the farm. There is testimony that she worked with exceptional energy and foresight so that the land improved and the farm became a model for the neighbourhood. She devoted much time to educating her sons and she also taught the maids and farm workers, down the years, so that most of them became literate and bilingual. The boys attended schools at Llangadog, Llanymddyfri and Abertawe (Swansea), and such an ambitious educational programme must have meant very considerable sacrifice on the part of their mother. She had had early on to endure grief and distress when she lost her only daughter; and later, at a very critical time she lost her eldest son at the age of twenty-nine, when he was a tower of strength on the farm, and when John was away from home at his studies. She continued farming until the age of eighty, and died in well earned retirement at Llandeilo seven years later, on 30th March 1895.

During these years she must have had time to reflect with quiet detachment on the tribulations and triumphs of a full life. The memory of the daily family prayers and the active participation of her sons therein, and their physical efforts in helping to build the small chapel near their home, would contribute to her serenity. No doubt she had moments of exultation when she recalled the excitement of Morgan returning home after being involved in the American Civil War; and finally, of course, she would re-live with mellow satisfaction the long triumphant professional progress of John, who was created a baronet a year before she died.

Although John's boyhood and days of youth were spent in Blaenllynant, he was actually born at his mother's old home, Beili, where she must have gone for her confinement. Beili still stands and the present occupier points out with pride the room, in the older back part of the farmhouse, where this remarkable boy was born on November 6th, 1840. In those days there were few avenues of 'escape' for '*plant y werin*', children of the country folk, but the one well-recognised gateway to a wider educational field of culture and experience—and it must be added social standing—was to become a minister of religion. John Williams may have cherished this ambition at one stage, for it appears that he undertook some local preaching engagements. This was the normal preliminary phase of preparation before being recommended for formal training at a theological college.

However, he must have changed his mind, because during 1857-8 he studied at Glasgow University, and in July 1859 he was accepted as an apprentice to two general practitioners in Swansea—Dr W. H. Michael and Dr Ebenezer Davies. Two years later, at the age of twenty-one he began formal medical studies at University College Hospital, London, and obtained his first qualification, L.S.A., in 1865, thereby joining a remarkable list of distinguished Welshmen who have been associated with that hospital. Some of these names deserve to be recalled with pride, and within a few years John Williams became eminently worthy of his place in that scintillating gallery of genius. In that gallery must be included the names of C. J. Blasius Williams, the grandson of Dafydd William, Swyddffynnon, who gave the first complete description of mitral stenosis, according to Willius and Dry; David Daniel Davis, of Llandyfaelog, one of the Welsh royal obstetricians, who delivered the Duchess of Kent when the future Queen Victoria was born; Timothy R. Lewis of Llangan, Pembrokeshire, one of the leading world figures in tropical pathology; Ernest Jones of Tregŵyr (Gowerton), who became one of the most eminent psychoanalysts in Europe; Sir Thomas Lewis of Glan Taf, near Cardiff, cardiologist, clinical scientist and ornithologist; and finally, Hugh Morriston Davies, who had links with Swansea (hence his name), a courageous pioneer in the field of thoracic surgery. The achievements of John Williams were destined to match, and in some ways to surpass, the contributions of these giants.

His first resident post was house surgeon at University College Hospital, and this was followed by posts as house physician at the Brompton Chest Hospital and Great Ormond Street Hospital for Children. During 1866 he obtained the M.R.C.S. and the M.B. (London), and he took the M.D. in the following year. He gained the M.R.C.P. (London) in 1873, and he was elected F.R.C.P. in 1879. There was an interesting and important phase in his early professional career when he returned to Swansea. It is not known whether this move was the reflection of a desire to practise in Wales, or that there were no suitable openings in London. He practised medicine at 13 Cradock Street for about five years, and it was during this period that he laid the foundation of his personal library. He married Mary Elizabeth Anne Hughes of Ynystawe in 1872 and soon afterwards returned to London, where he became assistant obstetric physician at University College Hospital. Nine years later he became full obstetric physician, and from 1887 to 1893 he served as the first Professor of Obstetric Medicine at the Hospital. He was President of the Obstetric Society in 1887. He was Physician Accoucheur to the Royal Family for many years, and it is probable his appointment was on the recommendation of Sir William Jenner, who was Physician to the Queen. In 1903 he retired from active practice and made his home at Plas Llanstephan, on the west side of the estuary of the river Tywi in his native county of Carmarthen. About seven years later he moved to Aberystwyth so that he could devote more time to guiding and encouraging the development of the National Library of Wales. He named his new home Blaenllynant.

John Williams' return to London co-incided with a momentous phase in the development of surgery, because this was the time when the principles of Listerism in the prevention and treatment of infection were being laid down, and Joseph Lister was appointed to the staff of King's College Hospital in 1877. Williams was an early convert and accepted the new teaching, and in fact found that it was already being practised when he took up his appointment in 1872. He soon became an enthusiastic supporter and practitioner of the new methods. According to Herbert Spencer ' it was due to his early employment of the antiseptic system that Williams largely owed his success in obstetrics and gynaecology '. In reporting the results of his early work in the field of midwifery, John Williams stated that ' there have been seven deaths in 1174 confinements (½ %) ', and on using corrosive sublimate instead of as at first carbolic acid and later potassium permanganate, he claimed ' since then we have had no death from Puerperal Fever, and an almost entire absence of mortality '.

Convincing success in this field gave Williams sufficient confidence to undertake abdominal surgery at a time when most of the senior gynaecologists were extremely reluctant to adopt such heroic measures. With great courage he embarked on pioneer work of a hazardous nature and of fundamental importance, especially in view of the heated controversies which developed as a result of the opposition of the more conservative ' non-operating ' gynaecologists. He has rightly been regarded as the first example of the combination of an expert obstetrician and a successful ' surgical ' gynaecologist, and this had far-reaching effects. Williams' success, as emphasised by Herbert Spencer, ' was the chief factor in obtaining for obstetricians the right to operate at the hospitals of other medical schools, a right now universally recognised, to the great advantage of gynaecology '.

As a clinician he combined accuracy of observation with maturity of judgement and courage to make decisions ; he assessed his results with detachment and honesty. (Some of his clinical case books are housed at the N.L.W.). It is said that he was not impressively eloquent as a public speaker, but he was effective and resolute. The list of his publications is not particularly impressive but he exercised his influence in other ways ; he was the first chairman of the *Journal of Obstetrics and Gynaecology of the British Empire*, and he was a very influential clinical teacher. The late Dr Hughes Jones of Swansea in his paper on Sir John Williams recalls a personal comment made to him in 1927 by Thomas Watts Eden—a distinguished pupil of Sir John—that his former ' Chief ' was ' the greatest teacher of his time '. In 1894, a year after retiring from his professorial chair, John Williams was created a baronet by Queen Victoria ; the K.C.V.O. followed in 1902, and in 1911 he was elevated to G.C.V.O.

During the thirty years of his professional life in London Sir John persisted, with sustained enthusiasm and superb judgement, in his determination to acquire a magnificent collection of rare Welsh books and manuscripts, and in this sphere too he was eminently successful. The acquisitiveness of book collectors is proverbial but in the case of Sir John his bibliophilic propensities did not amount to bibliomania. His motives were altruistic, because his life's dream was the creation of the National Library of Wales, and he devoted his wealth and leisure in pursuit of the realisation of his dream. He had a clear vision from afar of ' *tir yr addewid* '—the promised land, and it was a matter of more than forty years before he could, metaphorically, set foot upon it. For him that moment arrived in 1907 when the National Library was granted its charter. It is true that other distinguished Welshmen, for instance Sir Herbert Lewis in the political field, gave invaluable help ; it is also true that Sir John was wise enough to accept the guidance of literary friends like J. H. Davies, who later became Principal of the University College of Wales at Aberystwyth. Even so, the main credit for the creation of the National Library and its establishment at Aberystwyth belongs to Sir John Williams. (Plates 10 & 11)

Sir John Williams' academic stature outside Wales was recognised by the award of honorary doctorates of three Scottish universities—Edinburgh, Glasgow and Aberdeen. He was also honoured by the King of Denmark by being awarded the Grand Cross of Dannebrog. The University of Wales awarded Sir John an honorary doctorate of science in 1905.

In 1909 Sir John with a splendid gesture of magnanimity transferred his priceless collection of books, manuscripts, prints and drawings to the National Library. Included in Sir John's treasures was the Reverend Moses Williams Collection—a magnificent collection that contained nearly all the Welsh books printed between 1546 and 1742. Moses Williams, who was Vicar of Defynnog, a remote parish in the hills of Breconshire, was probably the most erudite cleric in Wales during the first half of the eighteenth century. He was a graduate both of Oxford and Cambridge, a Fellow of the Royal Society and indeed its temporary secretary at one stage, and he was on terms of close friendship with the most distinguished scholars in England. In addition to his extensive literary activities he was also indefatigable as a collector of rare books and copyist of old manuscripts. As a result of Sir John's foresight the collection was kept intact and safely preserved. By similar foresight he arranged to secure the unique Peniarth Collection which was in the possession of W. R. M. Wynne and his brother Owen S. Wynne. On the death of the latter in 1909 the collection came into Sir John's possession and he immediately donated it to the National Library. He was the first President of the Library and he continued to give his very generous support to it until his death in 1926 at the age of 86.

Sir John's keen awareness of his *Cymreictod* (Welshness) revealed itself in many other ways. He was one of the prime movers in the formation of the Welsh Hospital Unit that was sent out to South Africa at the turn of the century. Members of the Welsh Unit included such distinguished surgeons as Sir (later) John Lynn-Thomas of Llandysul, who temporarily gave up his consultant post on the staff of Cardiff Royal Infirmary to take charge of the Welsh Hospital in South Africa, and Professor Alfred W. Hughes, of Aberllefenni, who was released from the Chair of Anatomy at King's College, London. Alfred Hughes contracted typhoid on the voyage back and died soon after reaching home, at the age of thirty-eight.

Together with Dr Morgan Davies Sir John succeeded in detaching

Wales from the 'England and Wales Section' of *The Medical Directory* and thereby was able to gain some small measure of distinctive recognition for his fellow countrymen. (Dr Morgan Davies' letters are preserved with Sir John's papers at the N.L.W.) Furthermore, in conjunction with Sir Isambard Owen, he undertook an active part in the preliminary work of setting up the King Edward VII Welsh Memorial Association for the Prevention of Tuberculosis. The incidence of tuberculosis at that time was devastatingly high, 'the captain of the men of death' had deprived Wales of many of its illustrious sons and daughters while they were still young and with their early promise unfulfilled. This massive and imaginative new scheme proved to be an effective weapon in the control and cure of a disease that had ravaged Wales for a long time. The work of the 'Welsh Memorial', as it was affectionately known, attracted a great deal of attention throughout Europe and was widely acclaimed.

Such is the brief outline of the background and achievements of John Williams of Gwynfe. It is by any standards an extraordinary story of triumph over early disadvantages and misfortunes, an account of a life of enormous professional distinction and it is a unique record of enlightened generosity and benefaction. The Welsh nation will always remember him with deep affection and will remain for ever in his debt. At the same time special tribute must be paid to the memory of his widowed mother, Eleanor Williams, that splendid embodiment of the best features of '*diwylliant gwerin*', the culture of the country folk, of Carmarthenshire. Her intelligence and fortitude, her love of books, her well disciplined life and religious faith were the virtues that she gave to her son. On the sure foundation of that inheritance he built wisely and well.

And now I have left myself neither time nor space to continue with my appointed theme, namely, 'Introduction to Exhibition of Books and Manuscripts'. My dilemma has been resolved by the preparation of the printed Catalogue, in which all the items have been carefully documented, so that the Catalogue is something more substantial than a mere inventory of the exhibits. Here again Dr John Cule and myself received invaluable help from the staff of the National Library of Wales in the preparation and printing of the Catalogue. It is our sincere hope that members of the Congress will regard its contents as a helpful exposition of some of the treasures of our medical literature in Wales, and that it will prove to be of permanent interest.

BIBLIOGRAPHICAL NOTE

I owe a special debt of gratitude to my friends, Emeritus Professor Stephen J. Williams and Mrs Williams, who were present when this communication was given to the Congress. I had not realised until then that Mrs Williams was related to the Blaenllynant family. They kindly allowed me to borrow one of their treasured possessions—a copy of *Byr-Gofiant am Eleanor Williams*—and this small volume did much to illuminate the story of Sir John's early life. Much of this information has been included in this paper. Mrs Stephen Williams also showed me the cloak and bonnet which Eleanor was wearing in the photograph shown in that volume !

It is felt that a formal list of references is not necessary. Further information is available in *The Dictionary of Welsh Biography* about Sir John Williams, the Reverend Moses Williams and the Wynne family of Peniarth. There are further details about Sir John in *The National Library of Wales Journal*, Vol. I, pp. 173-232 ; and there is an interesting article on the medical aspects of his life by Dr Iorwerth Hughes Jones in Vol. IX, pp. 235-238 of the same *Journal*. The definitive work on the Reverend Moses Williams is the volume entitled *Bywyd a Gwaith Moses Williams*, by John Davies, (University of Wales Press, 1937). The comment on C. J. B. Williams is from *The History of Cardiology:* by Willius and Dry (Saunders, 1948). The standard volume on the history of the Library is *The National Library of Wales:* 1937.

ADDITIONAL BIOGRAPHICAL NOTE

It was after the completion of this paper that I saw the bilingual booklet, *John Williams* 1840-1926, by Ruth Evans. (University of Wales Press, 1952). It was evident that the author had seen a copy of *Byr-Gofiant*, and she had also drawn on other interesting source-material, including diaries, which enabled her to give a valuable kaleidoscopic picture of Sir John's life. The vignettes include a prophetic glimpse of him as a late teenage student at Glasgow. She also describes his deep awareness of his mother's financial sacrifice on his behalf, and after qualifying 'the first thing he did was to repay all she had spent on him.'

Perhaps the most delightful episode was that of John Williams converting his Gold Medal in Pathology into the wedding ring for his wife—and doing the job with his own hands ! It must have been a particularly hilarious occasion when his great friend, Marcus Beck, coming down from London to Swansea for the wedding, overslept and woke up at Carmarthen ! He was too late for the ceremony at Libanus Chapel, Morriston, but arrived in time to see the 'showers of rice and slipper '.

The booklet deals, of course, with more weighty matters as well, and the author has indeed provided a most admirable and comprehensive account ot the life and work of Sir John Williams.

Emyr Wyn Jones

DR ISAMBARD OWEN (1850—1927)

D. GERAINT JAMES

BACKGROUND EDUCATION

Herbert Isambard Owen was born on December 28th, 1850 at Chepstow, son of William George Owen, chief engineer of the Great Western Railway. His father had worked with the famous engineer, Brunel, whom he obviously admired for his son was named after Isambard Kingdom Brunel (1806-1859) who was also his godfather. They moved to live in Gloucester where he was sent to King's School, later Rossall, and in 1868 he entered Downing College, Cambridge (a college which later made him an honorary fellow). He joined St George's Hospital Medical School on 26th September 1871 and qualified M.R.C.S. (1875) and M.B., B.Chir. (Cantab.) (1876), thereafter staying at St George's to undertake junior hospital appointments, curatorship of the Museum, and becoming a consultant physician there in 1880. During this period he became M.D. (1882), F.R.C.P. (1885) and briefly a physician to Brompton Hospital (1883). His Cambridge M.D. thesis was entitled *The Treatment of Acute Rheumatism*. As a St George's Hospital medical registrar (1879-1880) he lived in Gloucester Gardens, but later as a consultant physician lived in 5, Hertford Street and at 40, Curzon Street, Mayfair. Miss Thackray told him that the Curzon Street house was the one described as Becky Sharp's in *Vanity Fair*. (Personal communication, Heulwen and Hedydd Isambard Owen).

PROFILE

He was six-foot in height, slim and rather frail in appearance, but nonetheless he had a deep melodious voice, and a Welsh power of oratory which alternated between deep emotion and light humour. He had a high forehead, Roman nose and a delicate chin (Plate 12). He was knighted in 1902 and soon after reaching Newcastle he married

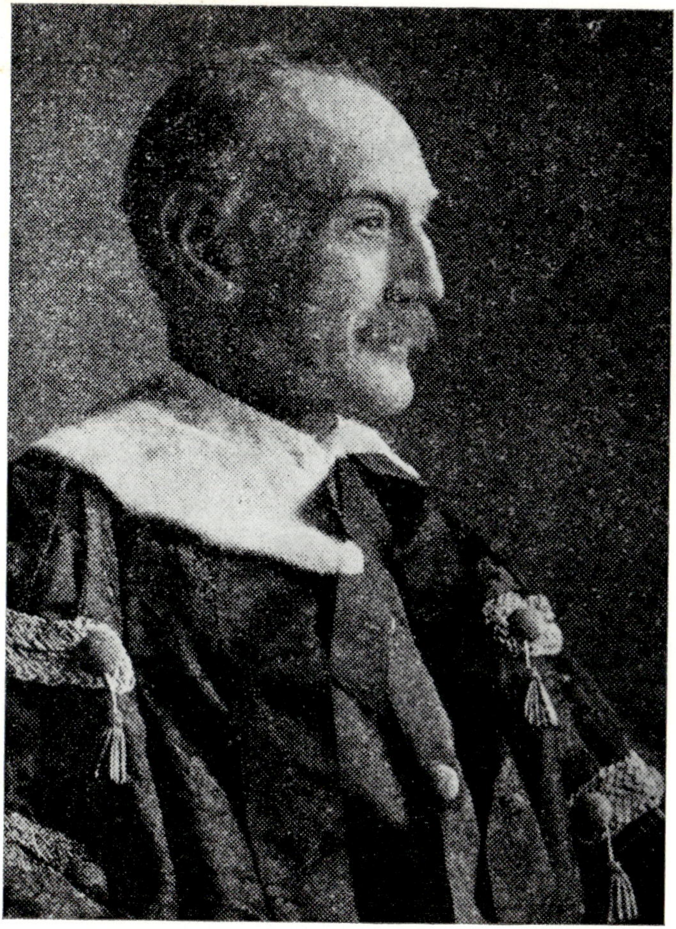

Plate 12
Isambard Owen

on 5th April, 1905, Ethel, daughter of the late Lewis Holland-Thomas of Caerffynnon, Merioneth, by whom he had two daughters, Heulwen and Hedydd.

He was an ardent Freemason, becoming Worshipful Master of the St Vincent Lodge, Bristol, and Senior Grand Deacon of the Province of Bristol.

He enjoyed cycling ; and pictures and music appealed to his Welsh artistry.

In view of his painstaking work, and skilful drafting of university charters, it is not surprising that he received honorary doctorates of the universities of Wales, Durham and Bristol.

He died suddenly in Paris on January 14th 1927, within a few hours of a stroke. His body was cremated at Père la Chaise Cemetery, Paris, and the ashes laid to rest in a grave near to that of his close friend, William Cadwaladr Davies, at Glanadda Cemetery, Bangor. (Jones 1967).

In an obituary in the *Welsh Outlook* (Defynnog James 1927) my father described his friend thus, '. . . His was a most charming personality. His charm seemed to me so overwhelming that if he had asked the King for Home Rule for Wales, His Majesty could not refuse his request. With keen and incontrovertible argument, with a suavity mixed with gravity, with an eye radiating kindness and keenness, he would overcome the strongest opposition, and make friends of his opponents. His magnanimity and sublimity (reflected even in the names of his daughters, Heulwen and Hedydd, who, with their beloved mother, today mourn their loss) relentless persistency, tact and resource, all combined to make him a successful diplomatist '.

I have recently found in the attic of my old Welsh home two group photographs of some historic interest for Isambard Owen and my father are seated together in the centre of the photographs. One of them was taken in Bangor in August 1904 during the course of ' Yr Ysgol Haf Coleg y Gogledd Awst 1af—13ef 1904 '. The other was taken in February 1913 at ' Cyfarfod Blynyddol Cymdeithas yr Iaith Gymraeg, Chwef. 1913 '.

UNIVERSITY OF LONDON

He was assistant dean and dean of the St George's Hospital Medical School (1884—1892) and lecturer in medicine (1899-1904) when he wrote a book on Materia Medica. He was a progressive perspicacious dean for he appointed Dr (later Sir) Patrick Manson as the first lecturer in tropical medicine in London, a position which Dr Manson held at St George's from 1895 until 1908. In 1897 he and Sir James Fowler drafted a scheme for the reconstitution of the University of London, which recommended a university of Westminster (Owen 1897). During Sir James Fowler's tenure of office as dean of the Faculty of Medicine of the University of London, Isambard Owen became vice-dean of this faculty from 1901 to 1904, until his move to Newcastle. After this move he was made honorary life governor of St George's Hospital (1905) fittingly in the year of his marriage.

During the London phase of his life he was also a most successful secretary (1881–1883) of the Medical Society of London, being largely responsible for the reconstruction of the society's premises.

His London Welsh connections were strong for soon after qualifying as a doctor he became a member of Council of the Cymmrodorion (1879), became president of the Welsh Language Society, and successfully drafted a charter for a new national Welsh university.

THE MEDICAL SOCIETY OF LONDON

Isambard Owen was elected junior honorary secretary on March 6th, 1882 becoming senior secretary on March 5th, 1883. The officers and council were pre-eminent members of the London medical profession of the day (Fig. 1) ; amongst these giants he proved a most successful secretary and on 1st December 1884, the president Arthur Edward Durham and his secretaries wrote a letter of appreciation '. . . In accordance with a resolution of the Council of the Medical Society of London we are desired to offer you this expression of their high appreciation of the exceptionally valuable services you rendered to the Society during your term of office as Honorary Secretary . . . The arrangements connected with the renewal of the Lease and the rebuilding of the premises entailed upon you a very unusual amount of work which was done most cheerfully and efficiently using your legal knowledge and architectural skill. The Council while offering you this expression of indebtedness to you ventures to add the hope that like success may attend you throughout your future career . . .'

He replied :— 'Gentlemen,

Permit me to assure you of my sincere appreciation of your very kind letter of the 1st inst. Though the business of the Society during my term of office made, I must admit, considerable

THE

OFFICERS AND COUNCIL

OF

THE MEDICAL SOCIETY OF LONDON.

ELECTED MARCH 6TH, 1882.

PRESIDENT.
FRANCIS MASON, F.R.C.S.

VICE-PRESIDENTS.

RICHARD QUAIN, M.D., F.R.S.
HUGHLINGS JACKSON, M.D., F.R.S.
ROBERT BRUDENELL CARTER.
J. CAWOOD WORDSWORTH.

TREASURER.
ALFRED WILTSHIRE, M.D.

LIBRARIAN.
WILLIAM H. ALLCHIN, M.B., F.R.S.E.

ORATOR.
E. SYMES THOMPSON, M.D.

COUNCIL.

C. THEODORE WILLIAMS, M.D. } *Chairmen.*
DAVID HENRY GOODSALL. }

HENRY FRANCIS BAKER.
R. S. FANCOURT BARNES, M.D.
SAMUEL BENTON.
WILLIAM HENRY BROADBENT, M.D.
SIDNEY COUPLAND, M.D.
JOHN HAMILTON CRAIGIE.
HENRY RADCLIFFE CROCKER, M.D.
THOMAS STRETCH DOWSE M.D.
JOHN HENRY DREW.
ARTHUR EDWARD DURHAM.
FREDERICK JAMES GANT.
HENEAGE GIBBES, M.D.
ALFRED PEARCE GOULD, M.S.
F. DE HAVILLAND HALL, M.D.
WILLIAM MILLER ORD, M.D.
WALTER PYE.
THOMAS GILBART-SMITH, M.D.
WILLIAM FREDERICK TEEVAN.

HONORARY SECRETARIES.

EDMUND OWEN.
ISAMBARD OWEN, M.D.

SECRETARY FOR FOREIGN CORRESPONDENCE.
SIR WILLIAM MAC CORMAC, D.Sc.

TRUSTEES.

Of the Real Estate.
FRANCIS HIRD.
CHARLES JOHN HARE, M.D.
THOMAS BRYANT.

Of the Personal Property.
CHARLES COGSWELL, M.D.
CHARLES H. F. ROUTH, M.D.
C. H. ROGERS-HARRISON.

THE ABOVE CONSTITUTE THE COUNCIL.

REGISTRAR.
WILLIAM E. POOLE.

VOL. VI. b

Fig. 1a. Officers and Council of the Medical Society of London 1882

THE

OFFICERS AND COUNCIL

OF

THE MEDICAL SOCIETY OF LONDON.

ELECTED MARCH 5TH, 1883.

PRESIDENT.

SIR JOSEPH FAYRER, K.C.S.I., M.D., F.R.S.

VICE-PRESIDENTS.

HUGHLINGS JACKSON, M.D., F.R.S. JOHN BRUNTON, M.D.
JOHN CAWOOD WORDSWORTH. ALFRED COOPER.

TREASURER.

ALFRED WILTSHIRE, M.D.

LIBRARIAN.

WILLIAM H. ALLCHIN, M.B., F.R.S.E.

ORATOR.

EDWARD LUND, F.R.C.S.

COUNCIL.

THOMAS GILBART-SMITH, M.D.
EDMUND OWEN.
} *Chairmen.*

HENRY FRANCIS BAKER.
SAMUEL BENTON.
SIDNEY COUPLAND, M.D.
JOHN HAMILTON CRAIGIE.
H. RADCLIFFE CROCKER, M.D.
JOHN HENRY DREW.
WILLIAM EWART, M.D.
JAMES KINGSTON FOWLER, M.D.
HENEAGE GIBBES, M.D.
DAVID HENRY GOODSALL.
GEORGE LAWSON.
HENRY MORRIS.
FRANCIS MASON.
EDMUND OWEN.
ARTHUR ERNEST SANSOM, M.D.
CHARLES BRODIE SEWELL, M.D.
THOMAS GILBART-SMITH, M.D.
WILLIAM HEATH STRANGE, M.D.
WILLIAM JOHNSON WALSHAM.
C. THEODORE WILLIAMS, M.D.

HONORARY SECRETARIES.

ISAMBARD OWEN, M.D. ALFRED PEARCE GOULD, M.S.

SECRETARY FOR FOREIGN CORRESPONDENCE.

SIR WILLIAM MAC CORMAC, D.Sc.

TRUSTEES.

Of the Real Estate.
FRANCIS HIRD.
CHARLES JOHN HARE, M.D.
THOMAS BRYANT.

Of the Personal Property.
CHARLES COGSWELL, M.D.
CHARLES H. F. ROUTH, M.D.
C. H. ROGERS-HARRISON.

THE ABOVE CONSTITUTE THE COUNCIL.

REGISTRAR.

WILLIAM E. POOLE.

Fig 1b. Officers and Council of the Medical Society of London 1883 demands upon the secretaries' time, I shall always look upon those two years with feelings of unmixed pleasure. I trust it may ever be my lot to do my work under such agreeable auspices and with such unexceptionable fellow-workers as the officers and fellows of The Medical Society of London '.

In keeping with tradition, he became vice-president at the end of his term as secretary. Had he stayed in London, he would also without doubt have become president.

During these years he made several case presentations on rheumatism, cardiac aneurysm, lardaceous disease, floating kidneys, and in 1904 he delivered the Annual Oration on ' The future of London Medical Education ' (Owen 1904).

UNIVERSITY OF WALES

Whilst still in consulting practice in London, Isambard Owen was already making decisive moves towards an integrated university of Wales instead of isolated university colleges at Aberystwyth, Bangor and Cardiff. In 1887 he organised a public conference which passed resolutions in favour of a national Welsh university with complete equality of the sexes. His draft charter prepared with Principal Viriamu Jones was accepted in 1893 by Welsh colleges, county councils and by the Intermediate Education Conference. It was approved by Parliament and passed under the Great Seal. He was appointed one of the Crown Members of the University Court, and in April 1894 he consented to act as honorary secretary until the statutes were completed and a registrar appointed.

In January 1895 the following appointments took effect :—

Chancellor : Lord Aberdare. Within a few weeks he died and was succeeded by the Prince of Wales (afterwards King Edward VII)

Vice-Chancellor : Principal Viriamu Jones

Senior Deputy Chancellor : Dr Isambard Owen

This was an office of considerable distinction for he was, in effect, the Prince of Wales' deputy (for the vice-chancellor, the academic head of the University was not the chancellor's deputy). As senior deputy chancellor, he had, in 1896, the honour of installing the then Prince of Wales as chancellor at Aberystwyth. His contact with the Prince of Wales at this stage was to serve him in good stead when he moved to Armstrong College, Newcastle, for King Edward and Queen Alexandra readily came to open the new wing of the college when he was principal there. He remained senior deputy chancellor from 1895 to 1910, during which time he also became president of the Welsh Language Society (1900) and helped Lord Davies of Llandinam to found the Welsh National Memorial Association against Tuberculosis—not surprising since Isambard had been (1883) consultant chest physician to the Brompton Hospital.

During 1916 he presented evidence to a Royal Commission on University Education in Wales which included the following :

Viscount Haldane (*Chairman*)
Hon. W. W. Bruce
Sir Owen M. Edwards
Sir W. H. Hadow
Sir A. D. Hall
Sir Henry Jones
Sir William Osler
Sir William Bragg
Miss Emily Penrose

His services as guide and counsellor to the university never ceased, for even at the time of his death in 1927 he was completing a draft scheme for a Welsh National School of Medicine.

NEWCASTLE-ON-TYNE (1904-1909)

In 1904 he gave up his London work to become principal of the Armstrong College, Newcastle-on-Tyne, arriving for the completion and official opening of the West front. Probably due to his personal influence, King Edward VII and Queen Alexandra combined this function with the opening of the new Royal Victoria Infirmary. When Isambard Owen joined Armstrong College, it was a relatively subordinate college. By the University of Durham Act (1908), Armstrong College and the Newcastle College of Medicine became equal partners with the Durham colleges in the administration of the university. This was a striking tribute to his diplomacy and organising genius.

UNIVERSITY OF BRISTOL (1909–1921)

In 1909 he was appointed vice-chancellor of the newly constituted university of Bristol, formed by the amalgamation of three institutions —a university college, a technical college and the old established medical school. Although by training a doctor, he strove vigorously to strengthen the faculty of arts in this university. He was the university representative on the General Medical Council (1910–1925) and became Senior Grand Deacon of the Province of Bristol.

In October 1912, he organised the installation of Viscount Haldane as chancellor with dignity and a flawless sense of ceremony. It was appropriate that he should receive an honorary LL.D. during the course of this installation.

G. A. Jones (1967) in his splendid M.A. thesis on Isambard Owen recounts the unbounded praise and respect of Sir George Oatley (1863–1950) chiefly known for his work (1912–1925) as architect of the university. Isambard Owen was no longer in office when the building project was finally completed but Oatley's letter is itself a monument of Isambard Owen's achievements for the university of Bristol—' You have had much more to do with the success of the building scheme than I have done. You have laid down what it should be and were the inspiration at its initiation. All that I have done has been to try to carry out what was in your mind. But honours rarely come to the right person. At any rate I am deeply sensible of what the scheme owes to you and it has been a grief to me that you could not be here to carry out its completion. At the top of the tower there is incised in the stone, out of sight of the ordinary observer, but for the gods to see and for all enquiring minds to discover if they will—

Φ TRIUMPHE

The i.o. is, of course, a play upon your name. It was Napier Abbot who gave me the idea years ago.

Yours very sincerely,

George H. Oatley.

CYMDEITHAS YR IAITH GYMRAEG
(THE WELSH LANGUAGE SOCIETY)

President : ISAMBARD OWEN
Secretary : DAVID JAMES (DEFYNNOG)

It was founded at the National Eisteddfod at Aberdare (1885) with a policy of introducing Welsh into the school curriculum . . . 'All members of the Society wish their children to acquire a sound knowledge of English but no harm will be done by nurturing the Welsh language which has been expected to die for a long time, but will live forever'. Their policy of academic bilingualism was entirely successful at the beginning of this century, for Welsh, as a subject, gained its first foothold in the State education system. It is a pity that it was allowed to lapse with the death of its president (in 1927) and its secretary (in 1928), within a year or so of each other. Had this first society survived, then it would probably have achieved its aims of three million bilingual Welshmen by 1984, and utilising the Welsh language in education to provide a more intelligent knowledge of English.

Although an English-speaking Welshman who spent nearly the whole of his life outside Wales, he was able to do more, and did more than many whose sole claim is that they have entered into the labours of others (Defynnog James 1927).

Again my father writes, '. . . He was the President and one of the founders of the Welsh Language Society. As its secretary for over 25 years, I had the pleasure of coming into personal contact with him on many occasions, especially after he left Newcastle-on-Tyne and came to Bristol. He would attend, at my request, small committee meetings in Cardiff, address large gatherings in the Rhondda, Pontypridd, and Carmarthen, fire the Welsh Summer School with enthusiasm, interview the Board of Education when necessary, and all this with grace, readiness and thoroughness. I had the pleasure of visiting him in 1921 at Weston-Super-Mare, and his kindness and that of Lady Owen on that occasion knew no bounds. He took me for a long walk up the hills behind Weston. While our eyes were feasting on the beauties of Somerset, he would relate, at my request again, the thrilling stories of the battles fought on behalf of Wales in London—

in the Lobby of the House of Commons and elsewhere (Defynnog James 1927).

The photograph was taken at the Annual Conference of the Welsh Language Society held that year in Newport in February 1913. At that time Isambard Owen had been president and my father secretary of the Society for about twelve years.

BRITISH MEDICAL ASSOCIATION

He was honorary secretary of the Metropolitan Counties Branch (1892–1897) and its representative on the Central Council of the B.M.A. (1896–1899) , and in 1895 he was local secretary of the large London meeting.

He had been secretary of the Section of Medicine at the Annual Meeting in Birmingham (1890), was vice-president of that section at the Annual Meeting at Nottingham (1892) and its president at the Annual Meeting at Swansea (1903).

He was a member of the Parliamentary Bills Committee from 1894 to 1897 and of the Medical Charities Commission from 1899 to 1902.

The B.M.A. decided to contribute to the advancement of clinical medicine by enlisting its members in the collection of clinical and epidemiological data. This was suggested by Professor (afterwards Sir) George Murray Humphrey in his presidential address at the Cambridge Annual Meeting (1880) and supported by Professor (afterwards Lord) Lister, Sir William Gull and Sir Wilmot Herringham. Isambard Owen became secretary of this Collective Investigation Committee which produced reports on centenarians (Sir George Humphrey), chorea (Sir Stephen Mackenzie) and cancer of the breast (Sir Henry Butlin). Isambard Owen also contributed with a report on diseases due to intemperance, which was published in the *British Medical Journal*, June 1888 and reprinted in the *Collective Investigation Record.* (Owen 1888).

EPILOGUE

Isambard died on 14th January 1927 and his wife, Ethel, on 15th June 1929, leaving two daughters, Heulwen and Hedydd Isambard Owen, who live together in north Wales since their repatriation in 1945 from occupied France. I wrote to them concerning my talk on their father to the Welsh History of Medicine Congress in September 1973 in Swansea. Their reply confirmed the warmth and respect that our fathers had for each other and they go on, '. . . We used to keep your photo on our schoolroom mantelpiece (wearing a white silk frock and a curl over your forehead !) with Nansi, Eurwen and Glesni—that was a few years ago. We have donated many things to Coleg Bangor. The Librarian came over last month to choose books and among others he eagerly seized on your father's delightful grammar for children—we used to love it as it was beautifully illustrated . . . Arthur Jones of the Normal College, Bangor lately produced an extremely comprehensive life of our father for his M.A. of the University of Wales. We have sent our copy to Bristol University . . . We too wrote father's life-story which was privately printed some years ago . . . our personal memories of our father as he was at home, and stories he told us about his childhood. It is now out of print, but all the Welsh Colleges have copies—' *Sir Isambard Owen*, by Heulwen and Hedydd Isambard Owen '.

Gwilym Arthur Jones' M.A. thesis (1967) is an outstanding work on the life and work of Sir Isambard Owen with particular reference to his contribution to education in Wales. I have obtained a copy which I plan to present to the Medical Society of London since Isambard's efforts in 1881 to 1883 were largely responsible for its reconstruction and survival, enabling us to commemorate its bicentenary in 1973 (James 1973).

REFERENCES

British Medical Journal (1927). Obituary. 1, 167.

James, Defynnog (1927). Obituary. *Welsh Outlook*, March 1927, p. 66.

James, D. G. (1973). 1773 and all that : bicentenary of the Medical Society of London. *New Engl. J. Med.*, 288, 1124.

Jones, G. A. (1967). The life and work of Sir Isambard Owen, 1850–1927. Dissertation in candidature for the degree of Magister in Artibus University of Wales.

Lancet (1927). Obituary. 1. 206.

Owen, Isambard (1888). Report on the inquiry into the connection of disease with habits of intemperance. *Brit. med. J.*, 1, 1309.

Owen, Isambard (1897). The schemes for the proposed Universities for London *Br. med. J.*, 2, 1869.

Owen, Isambard (1904). The future of London medical education. *Br. med. J.*, 1, 1177 and *Lancet*, 1, 1399.

Stephens, M. *The Welsh Language Today* (1973). Gomer Press, Llandysul.

EDWARD OSLER AND JOHN KEATS

ROBERT GITTINGS

This study celebrates briefly the curious conjunction, just under 160 years ago, of two doctor-poets at Guy's Hospital. One of these already has his eternal niche 'among the English Poets after my death', as his own words proudly prophesied. On Sunday 1 October 1815, John Keats, just under twenty years old, registered at the Counting House of Guy's Hospital for twelve months, and the following day paid his fees as a surgical pupil. He was an extremely promising pupil; for only four weeks later, he was accepted for the next vacant dressership, and on 3 March 1816, he re-registered for another year from that date, having become dresser to William Lucas junior. He went on to sit for the Society of Apothecaries examination, and obtained his licentiate on 25 July, becoming, in the words of the minutes of the Court of Examiners on that day, one of 'a class of well educated Practitioners', which the year-old Apothecaries Act of 1815 had been designed to foster. Something of Keats's achievement can be judged from the fact that the failure-rate in this year had been formidable; one student in nine had failed to satisfy the examiners, whether by previous qualification or by performance. The legend that the examination at that time was not a severe test, and that Keats succeeded largely through his classical ability to memorize the Latin terms in the *Pharmacopeia*, turns out to be a jealous invention, put about, long after Keats's death, by his then room-mate, Henry Stephens. Stephens went on to invent and give his name to the celebrated blue-black ink; but when he went up for this examination a few weeks after Keats, he failed. His chagrined belittlement of the qualification has caused many biographers of Keats to miss the fact of the latter's real medical ability.

Keats, however, already had ambitions as a poet, and was perhaps apt to overplay these 'amongst mere Medical students', as Stephens again somewhat jealously noted. He had, in fact, achieved publication in *The Examiner* of 5 May 1816, where his sonnet 'O Solitude' had been printed above the initials J.K. After his success in the examination, he arranged with his fellow-dressers to allow him to take time off for a period of summer leave. He went to Margate, already a popular seaside resort for the Londoner, and, avoiding the crowds, walked out to lonely places on the cliffs to write poetry, which painted

> The ocean with its vastness, its blue green,
> Its ships, its rocks, its caves, its hopes, its fears,—

He cannot have known that the cliffs where he sat had been themselves noted by another young poet and medical student, travelling in one of these very ships, on his way to London and to Guy's Hospital.

That summer, Edward Osler, a Cornishman, just over two years younger than Keats, had travelled by water from his native Falmouth, to enrol as a surgeons' pupil. He had already served his apprenticeship to a local doctor named Trevossa—the 'Corvosso' of the *Dictionary of National Biography* appears to be a misreading,—and he was already a poet with a modest reputation in his home town. In fact, he enlivened the voyage along the South Coast with a series of letters home, couched in quite poetic prose, about the beauties of the chalk cliffs, so different from the harsh granite of Cornwall. When he got to London however, the tune changed with the filth and crime, and noise of the big city. Osler wrote off a series of doggerel verses on the horrors of town life, and his letters for some time show him almost unable to adapt to what Keats, in his own letters, was just finding, on his own return to London, 'a beastly place in dirt, turnings and windings'; the two young Guy's men were showing similar reactions to the surroundings of their hospital in Southwark, then one of the most squalid quarters of London.

Keats's letters, however, show us nothing of the squalor of medical student life itself. The picture of the major poet's days in the dissecting room has always been drawn by biographers from the comparatively decorous pages of John Flint South's *Memorials*. In Edward Osler's letters, we have, for the first time, a realistic background to the work which was still Keats's major occupation, in his account of one of the freelance medical coach's dissecting rooms:

> On entering the room, the stink was most abominable. About 20 chaps were at work, carving limbs and bodies, in all stages of putrefaction, & of all colours ; black, green, yellow, blue, while the pupils carved them apparently, with as much pleasure as they would carve their dinners. One was pouring Ol. Terebinth on his subject, & amused himself with striking with his scalpel at the maggots, as they issued from their retreats ; here, were five or six who had served but a three years apprenticeship, most vehemently exclaiming against that regulation in the Apothecary's bill, which obliges every one to serve five years.

This letter also underlines the beneficial effect of the new examination of the Apothecaries Act. Intelligent students, such as Keats, who had served five years under Dr Thomas Hammond at Edmonton, and Edward Osler, with his five years under Trevossa, were to be the backbone of the new medical profession.

It is an irony, therefore, that these two young students at the same medical school, and sharing much the same tastes, never seem to have met, except perhaps in the casual rough-and-tumble of lecture-room and operating theatre. In those scenes, Osler certainly contributes to our knowledge of what medical life must have meant to Keats. He writes of incidents in the crowded theatre, where the patient became so terrified before a hydrocele operation—as well he might in pre-anaesthetic days—that he actually jumped off the table and fled from the room amid the hoots and jeers of the assembled student-audience. On the other side, as fellow-poets, there is actual concrete evidence that the young men both read and commented on the same works of literature, and in much the same manner. Early in December 1816, the fashionable Lord Byron brought out his narrative poem ' Darkness '. This was an extraordinary performance, a kind of doomsday exercise, imagining a world deprived totally of light, and, eventually, of life. At this moment, Keats was writing his own long and most successful early poem, ' Sleep and Poetry '. In a digression on the poets of his own day, Keats goes out of his way to castigate Byron for a poetry too sensational and horrible, even naming the name of Byron's own recently-published poem in these lines.

> But strength alone, though of the Muses born,
> Is like a fallen angel : trees uptorn,

Darkness, and worms, and shrouds, and sepulchres
Delight it ; for it feeds upon the burrs,
And thorns of life ; forgetting the great end
Of Poesy, that it should be a friend
To soothe the cares, and lift the thoughts of man.

At exactly the same time, Edward Osler was writing home with his estimate of Byron's poem. He too condemned it, but on slightly different terms from Keats's. Brought up as a Dissenter, though becoming in later life an Anglican hymn-writer, Osler knew his Bible thoroughly. He compared Byron's apocalyptic vision unfavourably with holy writ in the *Book of Revelation* ; and though he allowed the contemporary poet had power of expression and striking images, he could not find his picture, horrifying as it was, finally convincing. It is interesting that the two young men, one devoutly Christian, the other, Keats, already a free-thinker, both rejected Byron, not only on stylistic but also on moral grounds. Once more, one wishes there were evidence of their meeting and exchanging views.

Perhaps the final irony is that these two intelligent young doctors should both, after their training at Guy's and their good records there, give up medicine for literature. Keats's defection—if it may be called that—occurred at the point when each was writing his criticism of Byron. On 1 December 1816, Leigh Hunt, editor of *The Examiner*, whom Keats had recently met, published an article entitled 'Young Poets', praising Keats (and, with him, Shelley) and quoting in full Keats's sonnet 'On First Looking into Chapman's Homer', written in lodgings a stone's throw from the hospital. 'This', remarked Henry Stephens, 'sealed his fate'. Keats gave up going to Astley Cooper's lectures on surgery, and gave up all thoughts of the M.R.C.S., which everyone expected him to take next year. He told his astounded guardian, who had laid out nearly all Keats's small inheritance on a medical training, that he intended to devote his abilities to poetry. He ceased to be a member of Guy's on 3 March 1817. On that very day, his first book of poems was published. Four years later he was dead, having, in that short time, made himself 'among the English Poets'.

Edward Osler's career from medicine to literature was less dramatic. Obtaining his M.R.C.S., he served as resident house surgeon at Swansea Infirmary from 1819 to 1825. While there, he developed wide scientific interests, and in 1830 was elected Fellow of the Linnean

Society. The death of his much-loved first wife in 1828 seems to have permanently unsettled his medical career. As the result of a voyage as a naval surgeon, he published in 1830 a long poem, ' The Voyage ', with pathetic passages about his ' loved and lost Jennette '. Hymn-writing and local Cornish journalism occupied much of the rest of his life, though his best-known work is his *Life of Admiral Viscount Exmouth* (1835). A projected *Popular Introduction to Medicine* (1837) seems never to have been printed. A stained glass window in Kenwyn Church celebrates his death in 1863 ; but in the medical profession, he has his greatest celebrity as the uncle of Sir William Osler. It may well be thought that his greatest literary fame is to have been a hospital contemporary of Keats.

THE WELSH DOCTOR AS A POET

HENRY VAUGHAN—SILURIST

G. C. Davies

Henry Vaughan, the seventeenth century poet and doctor, appended the term Silurist to his name. Until recently its etymology has been derived from that romantic background beloved of the antiquarians. It was said that Locrinus, the son of Brutus, after his father's death, divided the lands of Britain between himself and his two brothers. After overcoming Humyr or Humber, Locrinus, the king of the Huns, found in one of the king's ships, three damsels of celestial beauty, one of whom was named Esyllt. She was to become associated with the country around the rivers Wye and Usk. Esyllt had a daughter by Locrinus, and her name was Hafren. She became immortalised in Môr Hafren, which is the Welsh name for the Severn Sea, in which both the mother and daughter were later drowned.

The Silures, first mentioned by Ptolemy, and later, by Tacitus, were the natives of the regions around the rivers Wye and Usk, including parts of Herefordshire, Monmouthshire, Brecknockshire, Glamorgan, and possibly, parts of Worcestershire and Gloucestershire. This name of Siluria however did not derive as the antiquarians believed from our story of Esyllt—whose name in Welsh records identifies it with Iseult—but more probably from a corruption of Seisyllwg.

The people of this area were a hardy and notable race, under the rule of puissant princes, both legendary and real, the most famous of whom was Caractacus, whose seat was said to be at Isca Silurum, now known as Caerleon, on the River Usk. This town is also held by some to have been the seat of King Arthur.

The patriots of this part of the country later became known as the Silurists, and one of the most famous of these was the seventeenth century poet-doctor, Henry Vaughan.

After a full life of medicine, poetic writing and Hermeticism, Henry Vaughan died at Llansantffraed and was buried in the little churchyard there, under a stone from Bwlch-yr-Arllwys quarry. Situated in a quiet corner of the churchyard, under a yewtree, on it can be seen that Henry Vaughan died in 1695, to be precise on St George's day, that same day of the year on which died Wordsworth and Shakespeare. The coat of arms on the stone is of the Vaughans of Tretower, consisting of a chevron between three boys' heads, each with a snake entwined about the neck. Some of the words on the stone are from Vaughan's poem, *The Mount of Olives*. They are also the last words of the earlier work, *The Tempest* by Herbert.

The only clue to the date of Vaughan's birth is given by the stone, which states that he died at the age of seventy-three. He must, therefore, have been born in either 1621 or 1622, most likely in the April of 1621, the elder of twin brothers at Trenewydd, or Newton St Bridget, in a house in the hamlet and manor of Scethrog, in the parish of Llansantffraed, in the hundred of Pencelli. The village is situated on the River Usk, and, nowadays, driving along the A40 from Abergavenny to Brecon, passing Tretower and Llangorse lake on the right, one journeys successively through Bwlch, Llansantfraedd and Scethrog, with Pencelli on the left.

Henry's younger twin Thomas was to become the famous mystical poet, Eugenius Philalethes. Also in the family was a younger brother William, and possibly an elder sister. Among the family's ancestors were people closely linked with the famous Herbert family, including two knights who had been slain at the battle of Agincourt, the first earl of Pembroke, the second earl of Worcester, and Sir Thomas Vaughan who makes an appearance in the third act of Shakespeare's *Richard III*, on his way to execution at Pontefract.

Little is known of Vaughan's childhood but he is believed, at the age of seventeen to have commenced studying, in the Michaelmas term of 1638, with his brother Thomas at Jesus College, Oxford. His brother completed the course, but Henry did not take a degree. There is no documentary proof of Henry ever having been at Oxford ; for example, there is no reference to him in the buttery accounts, a usually reliable source. He is, however, mentioned by the writer Wood in *Athenae Oxoniensis* and in the records of the Chancellor of Oxford as having been sued for debt by a local tradesman.

After two years reading 'Logicals', Henry was taken away by his father and sent to London where he is believed to have studied at the Inns of Court. Whilst there is no documentary proof that he did this, neither is there proof that Oliver Cromwell studied at Lincoln's Inn at the same time ; although the latter seems generally accepted as fact. Henry Vaughan was not called to the Bar.

From 1642 until the battle of Naseby on 14th June, 1645, Henry was a clerk to the judge, Sir Marmaduke Lloyd. He soon became a strong Royalist supporter but there is some question as to whether he actually fought in the war. He was possibly a lieutenant to Sir Herbert Price in the campaign of Chester, whereas his brother, Thomas was a captain in a Royalist Unit. Henry wrote in a poem in 1646 of being a captive at Raglan, which fell to the Cromwellian army on 19th August 1646, shortly before the end of the Civil War.

Following the end of the war, he returned home to settle down to writing poems and translating many important philosophical works.

Vaughan was fluent in Welsh and English, although he preferred to use the former. He must also have had a considerable working knowledge of Latin, Greek, German and French.

In 1646, Vaughan published a translation of Iuvenal's *Tenth Satyre*, along with fourteen other poems (registered at Stationers' Hall 15.9.1646). 1650 saw the publication of the first edition of *Silex Scintillans* (registered 28.3.1651). This was a volume of 122 sacred poems which Vaughan had written and compiled by the time he was twenty-two or twenty-three. A second part of this was published five years later in 1655.

The period of his life after 1650 was concerned with the writing of works relating to the establishment of the Puritan regime in Brecknockshire, and, also in 1651, perhaps Vaughan's most famous work was published, *Olor Iscanus, The Swan of Usk*. This book contained prose translations of works by Plutarch, Maximus of Tyre (a Greek Sophist), and Don Antonio de Guevara, Bishop of Cartagena. It is in two of these prose translations that Vaughan first shows a developing interest in medicine.

One of the Plutarch translations is *Of the diseases of the mind and the body*. This discusses the difference in these two types of disease and states that diseases of the mind are characterised by the patient wishing to flee from the physician. The treatise later compares diseases of the mind with storms at sea and tempests.

It is obvious from his choice of this work that Vaughan was not only becoming interested in medicine, but in the causes of disease, especially as related to the different schools of philosophy.

Another translation on diseases of the mind and the body, originally written by Maximus of Tyre (also known as Maximus Tirius) compares the two types of disease, equating the soul with a regent or king and the body with princes or subjects. It follows that as the regent is more powerful than his subject, the diseases of the soul must be more powerful or destructive than the diseases of the body.

In 1651 followed a collection of prose translations entitled *The Mount of Olives*, which includes works by Anselm, Archbishop of Canterbury. Following this in 1654, came a further collection, called *Flores Solitudinis*, and one year later the second part of *Silex Scintillans*. Completed at the age of thirty-four, after a serious illness and a religious conversion, this is vastly different from the first part, being very much concerned with metaphysics. The change may well have been due to the death of Vaughan's younger brother William, which had a profound effect on the writer. William died after a long illness following wounds in the civil war. The volume contains no less than five elegies to this brother.

In this second part of *Silex Scintillans* is a large number of references to medicine but all of which are to be found in earlier works by Donne or George Herbert, both of whom had been widely read by Vaughan.

It is not certain when Henry Vaughan first started to practise medicine, but he probably began a small rural practice late in the 1640's, in an area near Brecon. There is no evidence of when or where or even whether Henry Vaughan acquired a medical degree, but he was certainly styled as a physician after 1677 and had M.D. carved on his tombstone. The first mention of him as a physician is in the will of his daughter, Frances.

In those days there were many places at which one could obtain a medical degree but Vaughan does not seem to be mentioned at any of them. He is neither registered as having qualified at Oxford nor any of the other British universities including Dublin, nor is he registered at any of the Dutch universities including Leyden, nor at Padua. He is not on the roll of the Royal College of Physicians, nor is he recorded as having received a degree for services during the war. In those days one could obtain a medical degree from the archbishop of Canterbury, under a dispensation from Henry VIII, but Vaughan did not get one of these,—possibly because there was no archbishop from 1645 until 1660.

In 1673, Vaughan wrote to his cousin saying that his brother Thomas's employment was in physic and chemistry and added, ' My profession also is in Physic which I have practised now for many years with good success (I thank God), and a repute big enough for a person of greater parts than myself'.

By his first wife, Catherine, Henry Vaughan had one son and three daughters, and by his second wife, Catherine's sister Elizabeth, had another four children—again one son and three daughters.

In 1655 Vaughan published his most famous and medically important prose translation, *Hermetical Physick, or, the right way to preserve, and restore Health.* This is a book concerning physick based on the ' Principles of true *Philosophy* ', as was the ' Physick of *Hermes* '. The book is a translation of the work of Henry Nollius, also known as Nollyns or Nolles. Vaughan describes Nollius as a very reasonable and moderate Hermeticist and in his author's note, Vaughan writes, ' If any will be offended with this *Hermeticall* Theorie, I shall but smile at his frettings, and pitty his ignorance '.

The Hermeticists relate the causes of all diseases to the powers of philosophy, especially the astrological ones, so Hermeticism has been regarded as an esoteric religion, full of counter signs, fantastic beliefs and exotic rites, though based on doctrine and demanding spiritual preparation. They thought, for example, that whereas some diseases were caused by gods, others were caused by fire, and that pregnancy was due to impregnation by a star.

Perhaps the most famous of the Hermetical Physicists alive at the time was Henry's brother, Thomas. He died in the year of the great fire of London and his death is recorded in true Hermetical fashion. He was staying at the house of the rector of Albury when ' as twere suddenly when he was operating strong mercurie, some of which by chance getting up into his nose marched him off'.

The Hermetical Physicians believed that they could cure diseases which the Galenists could not, such as leprosy, gout, and some of the epilepsies.

The basic message of Hermetical Physick is the prevention of disease for which several suggestions are put forward including :

Lead a pious and wholly righteous life.
Follow after sobriety.
Eat not greedily and drink not immoderately.
Eat simple foods.
Eat only one type of food and drink at each meal.
Eat only foods to which you are used.
Use antidotes freely.
Change habitation if the air is contagious.
Use not too frequently the permissions of marriage.

The remainder of the treatise deals with the preparation of medicines and introduces medicines made from metallic sources, in preference to the earlier herbal medicines, being a consequence of the Hermeticists' interest in chemistry and metallurgy. The book concludes with a short discourse not only on the correct behaviour of the physician, but also of his patient when undergoing a course of physick.

Vaughan was attracted to the Hermeticists by their principle not to accept anything at its face value, but to criticise even the most accepted of theories by testing it with experiment. He was convinced that to be a successful physician one must be addicted to no particular school, but must be prepared to learn from all.

The last of Vaughan's works was *Thalia Rediviva*, published in 1678 and containing a poem 'Daphnis' in which is a description of the portal vein.

In 1695 Vaughan died. The man is, probably best summed up by one of his biographers, Miss Guiney, who wrote: 'One can picture him on his hardy Welsh pony, drenched in the mountain mists, close-hatted, big-cloaked, riding alone, and looking abroad with those mild eyes which were a naturalist's for earth and sky, and a mystic's for the spiritual world'.

The final accolade was given in the poem of 1928 by Siegfried Sassoon: 'At the Grave of Henry Vaughan' from *The Heart's Journey*:

Above the voiceful windings of a river
An old green slab of simply graven stone
Shuns notice, overshadowed by a yew.
Here Vaughan lies dead, whose name flows on for ever
Through pastures of the spirit washed with dew

And starlit with eternities unknown.
Here sleeps the Silurist ; the loved physician ;
The face that left no portraiture behind ;
The skull that housed white angels and had vision
Of daybreak through the gateways of the mind.
Here faith and mercy, wisdom and humility
(Whose influence shall prevail for evermore)
Shine, And this lowly grave tells Heaven's tranquillity
And here stand I, a suppliant at the door.

REFERENCES

1 Nicholas, Thomas (1874). *The History and Antiquities of Glamorganshire.* London. Reprint, 1970 (Stewart Williams), p. 24.
2 Wood, A.à. (1721). *Athenae Oxonienses,* 2nd ed., Vol 2, p. 926. B. Knaplock, *etc.,* London.

BIBLIOGRAPHY

Bennett, Mrs. J. (Frankau) (1953). *Four Metaphysical Poets ; Donne, Herbert, Vaughan, Crashaw,* 2nd ed. Cambridge University Press, Cambridge.
Hutchinson, F. E. (1947). *Henry Vaughan, a life and interpretation.* Clarendon Press, Oxford.
Mahood, M. M. (1950). *Poetry and Humanism.* Cape, London.

THE WELSH POET AS A MEDICAL HISTORIAN

GLYN PENRHYN JONES

The supreme genius of the English language proclaimed that 'the lunatic, the lover and the poet are of imagination all compact', and it is clearly difficult to define a poet or bard, versifier or rhymster. The Poet Laureate has been described as a mere 'Versifier Royal' and his office has included such notables in their own way as Alfred Tennyson, Alfred Austin, C. Day-Lewis and John Betjeman. Not only are we in difficulty in defining 'a poet', but doubly so in the term 'Welsh poet'—be he again *prydydd, bardd* or *rhigymwr.* The world at large generally assumes that Dylan Thomas was a Welsh poet—after all *he was Welsh* and *he was a poet.* So were Henry Vaughan, George Herbert, Vernon Watkins, Alun Lewis and even Edward Thomas, but they chose to write in English—their medium and their message was English, and thus they were essentially English poets and were virtually outside the Welsh literary and poetic tradition. I know that the Scots would hardly consider Robert Burns to be a Sassenach poet (he did write in English)—perhaps they would compromise by calling him a Lallans poet, or more non-committally in the meaningless term, a 'British' poet. And then again was Yeats an Irish poet, when his fame as a poet rests on his English poetry, and what about Hilaire Belloc who wrote English poetry but who was of a mixed French-Irish ancestry ? There is no difficulty about calling Richard Wilson a Welsh painter or Alan Ramsey a Scots painter or Benjamin Brittain an English composer, but when the medium of artistic expression is the spoken or written word in a language, then we must surely confine the term 'Welsh poet' to those who use the medium of the Welsh language.

That language (as you now know, I trust) is one of the oldest living languages of Western Europe, and the earliest examples of its poetry date from the sixth century ; it is truly remarkable that those ancient sixth century epics are comprehensible to the educated Welshman of today. Beowulf, the Anglo-Saxon epic, dates from the eighth century but is basically Germanic and now reads like a foreign tongue. If English literature, as we now know it, began with Chaucer, then Welsh literature in comparison is of a hallowed antiquity indeed. At least over the fourteen centuries of its tenacious if now tenuous existence, Welsh poetry—apart from its inherent artistic values and beauty—abounds with social commentaries, reflecting the political and cultural evolution of Wales in the manner of all national literatures. And even more so *in Wales*, since the poet here has always enjoyed the sympathy and the acclaim of his fellow countrymen to a far greater extent than in England. He in his turn has been ever ready with the judgements, praises and castigations that have been expected of him.

The internal evidence of some poetic compositions sheds light on the poets' own infirmities, and secondarily on the current concepts of diseases and their incidence. We know, from the format of their paintings, that Cézanne, Renoir, Pisarro and Degas were all myopic, that El Greco was astigmatic, and that John Constable was partially colour-blind. The ebb and flow of William Cowper's and John Clare's poetic geniuses indicate their manic-depressive state—episodic melancholia was a common eighteenth century affliction. Some of their contemporaries in eighteenth century Wales followed the same clinical fashion, Lewis Morris and Ieuan Fardd, both suffered from hypochondria, 'the spleen'. William Thomas (Islwyn), the poet of Gwent, followed suit in the nineteenth century and with him a whole corpus of mid-Victorian Welsh versifiers, obsessed with death, in the manner of John Donne, and generally referred to as the 'Cemetery School'. The fashionable addiction to laudanum in the early nineteenth century influenced the poetry of Coleridge and the prose of De Quincey ; it also kindled the fervid imagination of Iolo Morganwg, the 'onlie begetter' of the Gorsedd of the Bards at the National Eisteddfod of Wales. These poetic trends reflected the current climate of opinion and the cultural *mores* of the time, and have their parallels in English and Welsh poetry. Again, the physical infirmities of the bards, may have contributed to their inspiration ; it is conceivable that Byron's talipes equinovarus influenced his political and poetic heroics, that Pope's spinal deformity contributed to his waspish epigrammatic quips. In Wales we are historically fortunate in that the character and the physical peculiarities of the bards were often evident in their names and epithets ; to distinguish all the Joneses and Thomases of today we must have Jones the Milk and Thomas the Tax, and they have their poetic counterparts for Gruffydd Gryg, the sixteenth century Welsh poet was evidently *cryg*, a stammerer. Presumably both the 'Gwargam' and Dafydd Gam had congenital kyphosis. Llefoed Wynepglawr had the flat face of lupus, syphilis or leprosy ; Ithel Grach presumably suffered from an exfoliative disease, possibly psoriasis.

But we must turn to the poems themselves—the vast majority of them in the systematised alliterative verse, *cynghanedd*, that has characterised Welsh poetry from the beginning—for the eclectic facts of interest to the medical historian. The earliest of these, in general, would only excite the military medical historian, referring as they do to the nasty, brutish, and short lives of the peasantry in tribal society. The Anglo-Saxon '*Maldon*' poem of the tenth century, the French '*Chanson de Rolande*' of the eleventh century, and the Icelandic sagas, all have common ground with the early Welsh epics of Aneurin and Taliesin and others of similar vintage. Deaths in battle are commonplace, entrails hang festooned on gorse bushes, '*Angeu a gawsant a mynych goddiant*' (Death they have suffered and frequent pain). Heads are cut off by the hundred ('*Vi a leddis cant pen*'.) But among these insistent sanguinary pageants one encounters the occasional gem such as the picture of ageing, which must have been an uncommon experience in those days, in the Llywarch Hen poems of about the seventh century. In a picture reminiscent of a Dürer engraving an old man admits '*wyf cefngrwm, wyf trwm, wyf truan*'. (I am bent, heavy and wretched) and his *pedwar prif casbethau* (his four great hates) are '*pas, henaint, haint a hoed*' ('a cough, old age, disease and longing'). His back is bent like his old wooden crook ('*baglan bren*'). He is the Lear of Shakespeare.

A sequence of stanzas in this poem are recited by a *claf* of Abercuawg (The sick man of Abercuawg.) One writer has suggested that he was a leper—at least his affliction appears to have kept him from the battlefield—perhaps the only blessing of his dreaded leprosy. The prevading belligerence of the pre-Norman Welsh can be surmised from the fact that the Chronicles of the Princes, *Brut y Tywysogion*, record that between 949 and 1046 no less than 35 Welsh rulers died by violence, a further four being blinded. One entry for 1043 records that Hywel ab

Owain, king of Glamorgan, died in 'his old age', a demise so uncommon apparently as to deserve a special mention in this record of the monastic scribe.

But it was not war and pillage and the occasional catastrophic harvest in that very vulnerable society of early mediaeval Wales that decimated lord and labourer alike (*gwych a gwachul*). Always menacingly poised was the fourth horseman of the Apocalypse, pestilence. And Welsh poetry throughout the period of the Princes and right up to modern times was eloquent in lamentation and despair on the depredations of the traditional epidemics.

The true nature of some of these epidemics is often a matter of conjecture and controversy. Professor Shrewsbury has questioned the nature of the Plague of the Philistines, hitherto generally accepted as a classical visitation of bubonic-pneumonic plague. (It seems indeed that nothing is sacred). Since contemporary descriptions of the ancient epidemics are notoriously imprecise and unspecific, and speculation on their nature is inevitable, a gentle academic jousting is enjoyed by all. Allusions in Welsh literature to pestilential disease are likewise frustratingly vague, poetically bedecked perhaps, but clinically bare. Time and again the medical historian in this field is much like the clinician trying to sort out the symptoms of a patient who just will not stop talking. There are several instances in Welsh mediaeval poetry, in the *cywyddau* of the poets of the princes and the later schools, where the manifestations of disease as presented are so protean and so osbcurantly verbose that the affliction could be anything in the spectrum between devastating plague and mass hysteria. However some *cywyddau* leave no doubt about the diagnosis and this is particularly and poignantly true when the poet himself is the immediate eye witness of the cataclysm, when his own family was threatened, and when his own children died in consequence.

There were episodic outbreaks of bubonic plague in Wales throughout the fifteenth century—in the wake of the mid-fourteenth century European pandemics ; those episodes of '*haint y nodau*' (the infection of the lymph-nodes') are vividly recorded in the *cywyddau* of those Welsh poets who suffered personal tragedies. Ieuan Gethin ap Ieuan Lleision—although some manuscripts ascribe the authorship to Llywelyn Fychan ap Llywelyn Foelrhon—lost five children from the disease, firstly one Ifan, then another Ifan nine years later at the same time as the deaths of Dafydd, Morfudd and Dyddgu. There is little doubt what killed them ; their father bewailed the *swllt mewn cyswllt cesail*—' the deadly shilling in the depth of the armpit ' ; ' glands like little onions here and there, as dangerous as hot embers, inch-long harbingers of death '. And then the haemorrhagic black rash, ' seeded like black peas, spread like sea-coal '. ' *Galar oedd im eu gweled* ' he cried, ' I grieved to see them '.

Similar outbreaks no doubt caused the deaths of the ten children of Gwilym ap Sefnyn, a north Wales poet of the mid-fifteenth century. Dafydd Llwyd o Fathafarn, of mid-Wales, about 1440—1450 described the death from the plague of the girl he loved in a memorable *cywydd*, uniquely combining the poet's lament with a remarkable clinical objectivity. ' *Ysgrifen chwarren a'i chwŷs yn llywio dan ei llewys, A hefyd i gyd ei gwar dimeiau fel nod mwyar* '. ' The graphic gland, the trailing sweat, under her sleeve, Mites like berries around the nape of her neck '. The rash he described as ' powdered ermine on a lovely white skin ', as ' brown pepper and ink on white paper '. These English paraphrases are mundane compared with the Welsh original, but even these make us ruefully aware that the phraseology of our current medical textbooks is pretty insipid and humdrum.

Dafydd Nanmor, another north Walian, described an epidemic with similar clinical features in 1448 (possibly 1478), and Tudur Aled, later in the fifteenth century, described how a nobleman of Flintshire and his family died of ' the black rash ' (' *Y Frech Ddu* '). In the sixteenth century Gruffydd ab Ieuan ap Llywelyn Fychan, of St Asaph, again in *cywydd* form, described a Denbighshire outbreak of bubonic plague—either the 1535 or the 1557 visitation to Shropshire and the other Border counties—' *Gwenwyn yw'r bel lle y delo ; Saeth y farwolaeth yw fo* '—' The bubo is poison wherever it comes ; It is the arrow of death '. The threnody of Ieuan ap Madoc ap Dafydd about his fellow poet Syr Dafydd Trefor in the fifteenth century ' *Gwae o'r nod ddyfod a'i ddwyn* ' (' Woe that the bubo wrested him away ') certainly refers to bubonic plague. It seems that Robin Ddu ap Siencyn Bledrudd o Fôn, Gruffydd Dwnn, Rhisiart ap Rhys, Lewys Morgannwg, and Ieuan ap Rhys ap Llywelyn, all fifteenth or early sixteenth century poets, were aware of the decimations of bubonic plague. There is no doubt therefore that in that golden era of Welsh *cynghanedd* poetry, the ubiquitous plague often fired the poetic imagination.

Smallpox likewise ; the Welsh poet often remarked on the pock-marked faces of so many of his countrymen. Tudur Aled, at the turn of the sixteenth century, when smallpox was commonplace, described the arms of a buckler-shield—perforated as if by smallpox—(‘*A'i freichiau oll o'r Frech Wen*’). His contemporary Lewys Môn described an old pitted mill stone as pock-marked. Many of the popular lyrics and ballads of eighteenth century Wales referred to the *frech wen*, its deadliness and its disfigurments. One of the peasant bards of the 1730's, Cadwaladr Roberts of Pennant Melangell, bewailed his own fate in verse after an attack of smallpox and more particularly of his damaged matrimonial prospects, obviously pock-marked and very repugnant to the pretty maidens ; thus, only hags for him for ever more ! No doubt he was voicing the fears of many of his kind before the advent of variolation and vaccination in these islands.

The bards were naturally reluctant to record their venereal vicissitudes, and latter-day academics still more reluctant to give them light of day. Indeed for such gems of socio-medical *mores* it appears that one has to delve into an obscure volume entitled *Welsh Aedoeology* published in Germany, with a most unlikely editor, one Egerton Grenville Bagot Phillimore. However Dafydd Llwyd o Fathafarn, the author of the moving elegy to his lady who died of the plague, himself contracted gonorrhoea, and waxed just as eloquently about that infection, apparently widespread at that time, about 1450. He admits though, as a loyal Welshman, that the infection was acquired in England. One or two of the rumbustious, if not Rabelaisian, Welsh poets of the eighteenth century, Lewys Morris and Thomas Edwards (Twm o'r Nant) did imply that venereal infection was quite prevalent. In fact, a bardic and bucolic colleague of Twm o'r Nant, Dafydd Samwell, an alcoholic and a laudanum addict, naval surgeon and no mean poet himself, accompanied James Cook to the Pacific and there witnessed the death of his Captain. He published, in 1786, *A Narrative of the Death of Captain Cook and Observations respecting the Introduction of the Venereal Disease into the Sandwich Islands*—the result of his own meticulous observations on the social habits of the British tar in the South Pacific at that time.

In the immediate pre-industrial period of British history, several Welsh poets, particularly the ballad-mongers, recorded many of the more significant socio-medical events. The late 1720's were notorious years of death in many parts of Wales. Deaths were commonplace, with the rural parish records providing a clear testimony for the ravages of famine and of famine fever, typhus. One ballad writer of

Bodedern, Anglesey, signally described the morbid years of 1728-29 in that locality. Again in the year 1740-42 typhus and ' bloody flux ' added havoc to the general destitution, a morbid combination well known to the rustic poets of the period in Wales. Commentaries in verse, for popular edification, on similar catastrophies continued well into the twentieth century, being evocative and not only on the socio-medical milieu of expanding industrial south Wales, but also recording such visitations as the four major cholera epidemics between 1832 and 1866 and the typhoid outbreaks of the 1870's.

But one of the foremost causes, in fact, the single major cause of death in nineteenth century Wales was tuberculosis, and to the Victorian Welsh poet this was manna for the muse. During the middle years of the nineteenth century some three thousand people, mostly young, were dying annually of phthisis in Wales and the mortality rate here fell some twenty-five years after it had started to fall in England in the 1850's. As many of the deaths occurred in children and since the disease was so widely morbid both in rural Wales and in the industrial south and north-east many of the vernacular poets of the period testified, often from harrowing personal experience, to the banes and perils of consumption. J. R. Pryce (Golyddan), a medical apprentice, died of tuberculosis in 1862 when the disease was it its zenith of morbidity in Wales.

He was an introspective romantic and had modelled his poetry and his life on that of Keats, likewise following him in death. His Gwenonwy, who figures in his epic poem to Death, is directly comparable to ' *La Belle Dame . . .*' As a potential doctor, and as a prolific poet, although in a different plane of sensibility, his career parallelled Keats remarkably ; but Golyddan was essentially a Victorian who was overwhelmed with the idea of death, at a time when death was commonplace, and in that respect he was no different from Tennyson, Christina Rossetti, Coventry Patmore, and other English contemporaries.

Welsh ballads of the late seventeenth century referred to the malevolent consumption ; some poets of that period list the clinical signs of disease in a way that leaves no doubt about its nature. Robert ap Gwilym Ddu, one of the most distinguished of the strict metre poets in Wales in the nineteenth century described the death of his only daughter from tuberculosis in 1834 in a *cywydd* of the classical mould. There seems no doubt that she died of pneumonic phthisis. The heavy debilitating and deadly cough, the drenching sweats, the toxic flush are all noted meticulously by the grieving father. The poetic form was the same, the familiar tradition was the same, as in medieval Wales, but the disease now was pneumonic phthisis and not pneumonic plague.

A little later, Elis Wyn, another poet of Gwyrfai, a notorious black spot for tuberculosis until now, saw his sister die of the disease, as he must have seen many others. He noted the lassitude, the pallor, the weakening voice, the beady brow of the advanced tuberculous patient. Between 1840 and 1880 a whole array of young Welsh poets died of tuberculosis ; the deaths of so many promising young men is a stark reminder of social conditions in the towns and villages of mid-Victorian Wales.

This however was the last of the great pestilences, those catastrophies that caused the poet in Wales to voice the fears of the peasant. It is symptomatic of our history and of our nation that the Welsh poet of today, as our current Eisteddfodau confirm, is now concerned with the modern plagues of biological, chemical and cultural pollution. In this he is again a mirror of his generation ; he may only protest plaintively about the growth of the subtopian Sahara but he is one of the breed that Shelley once called ' the unacknowledged legislators of the World '.

This paper was read by Glyn Penrhyn Jones at Swansea on 7th September, 1973. Because of his untimely death shortly afterward it was retyped incorporating his marginal notes, and otherwise needing only minor corrections, with the help of Emyr Wyn Jones.—*Editor.*

THE INTERACTION OF WAR AND PLAGUE IN THE LATER MIDDLE AGES[1]

RALPH A. GRIFFITHS

Of all the horrors associated with the Vietnam War, the intrusion of plague is one of the most grievous. At times, the seering impact of war on Vietnamese society in the mid-twentieth century has been exacerbated by the interaction of war and plague in a sector of the globe where plague is still active and endemic.[2] So much greater was the impact of these two phenomena on western Europe in the later middle ages. In the fourteenth and fifteenth centuries, they afflicted a much wider geographical area, a much larger population, and a population that was much less well prepared medically for the onslaught of both. And they did so over a much longer span of time. As a result, the countries of western (as opposed to eastern) Europe shared a common, debilitating experience in these centuries.[3] Indeed, war and plague together are arguably the two most potent factors determining the evolution of contemporary European society.

Warfare cast a larger shadow over western Europe in the later middle ages than at any time since the Viking assaults half a millennium earlier. In the first place, states were at war with one another ; England and France, for example, fought each other almost continuously for more than a hundred years. Secondly, countries were racked with internal stife ; France's political rivalries, for instance, burgeoned into several civil wars. And, finally, urban and rural uprisings touched the humblest inhabitant of a city like Florence and a countryside like that of the Beauvaisis, to the north of Paris.[4] To claim for the twentieth century a novel concept of ' total war '[5] is to forget that such a concept is a relative one. Wars in other ages (and war-torn late-mediaeval Europe especially is one of these) had for those living through them just as direct and terrifying an impact ; indeed, in the case of the fourteenth and fifteenth centuries, they probably enveloped many more people than wars had done hitherto.[6] In the warfare of the later middle ages larger numbers of men were involved than ever before. They were drawn from wider social spectra, and not only served themselves under arms (and with arms that were becoming more accurate and sophisticated in their destructiveness and capacity for maiming and killing), but were also required to support the combatants with food, supplies, money and weaponry.[7] And they did so for longer periods at a stretch than had hitherto been common.[8]

This was the very era that witnessed onslaughts of endemic plague of unique intensity and magnitude in the recorded history of western Europe.[9] Whatever the current disputes about the capacity of medieval plague to kill (and they range from an over-modest 5 % to incredible contemporary estimates which amount to more than 100 % !), there can be no doubt that it induced an unusually high incidence of death.[10] What is more, it recurred again and again after its first appearance in the west in 1347, frightening and debilitating Europeans and ravaging a population that was medically defenceless and already experiencing serious nutritional problems.[11]

Historians have long been assiduous in examining the nature of this plague, utilising—perhaps over-utilising—the sadly innumerate statements of contemporary writers and chroniclers. More recently, they have been ingeniously bending imperfect statistics of appointments of clergy, records of wills and registrations of lawyers, tax assessments, the deaths of earls and bishops, figures of declining rents, and the rest, to serve as a mirror of the plague attacks.[12] For simply the size of the death-rate is one of the most vexatious problems of late-mediaeval historiography. Historians have been slower to turn their attention to the effects of war, but the so-called Hundred Years' War between England and France is now having its costs estimated, its campaigns examined, its combatants (particularly their leaders) scrutinised, and even the mass of non-combatants investigated selectively for their reactions to the war and their fate in wartime.[13] It is an investigation still in its infancy. Hardly begun is the much more difficult task of assessing the joint, and often simultaneous, impact of war and plague on late-mediaeval society—what the French would rather grandly call *conjoncture*. To isolate the effects of either one or the other is necessary, but in many communities in western Europe, whether in the wheat fields of Caldicot in south-east Wales or in the vineyards of the Bordelais in France, to be content with such isolated studies runs the risk of misrepresenting the impact of both and oversimplifying the complexities of historical explanation. To apportion responsibility between war and plague in satisfying proportions is well nigh impossible with the scanty statistical evidence available from the fourteenth and fifteenth centuries, but the art of impressionistic historical reconstruction can come close to a convincing reality.

The weight of the impact of war and plague on communities can be illustrated by one simple example. Cheshire in the mid-fourteenth century received constant calls from its lord, Edward, the Black Prince, to provide men (especially archers) for his armies going to France. Their uniforms, arms and equipment were largely paid for out of local Cheshire revenue. Hundreds of Cheshiremen fought at Crécy in 1346; in 1355 400 archers were summoned, with reinforcements to follow during the next year; in 1359 another 400 Cheshiremen were called out, and in 1363 yet a further 200.[14] And these were in addition to those men who were raised and equipped privately by other lords in the county. It all amounted to a substantial burden on the local population—and one which the county was called upon to shoulder only a few years after the arrival of the plague in Cheshire in 1348. In that year alone the abbot of Chester died of the disease, and so did the prioress of St Mary's, the prior of Norton, and at least twenty-four clerics in charge of Cheshire parishes. On the manor of Drakelowe alone, fifty-seven males died in 1348, and over a much wider area houses were left vacant, rents collapsed, and the land was deserted of its tenants.[15] Such could be the starkly obvious, but nevertheless profound, impact of *conjoncture*.

Contemporaries saw the consequences of war and plague merge in their own experience, and some of them were aware of the importance of *conjoncture*—and said so. Historians can do no better than take their cue from such writers. Take the five sole remaining 'good men' (*cinq bonnes gens*) of the parish of Vignolles in Gascony who packed their bags and left their homes to go and live in the city of Bordeaux at the beginning of the fifteenth century. They decided to move from their locality because, they said with deep resignation, 'of the mortalities and the war which have lasted a long time and which still continue'.[16] Or consider the plight of Montpellier in south-eastern France by 1376; with understandable hyperbole, the duke of Anjou commented in that year that 'the population, which is scanty enough owing to mortalities and epidemics that have flourished in these parts, and also to wars wherein many have perished, may be diminished to the greatest possible extent, and the world brought to nothing . . .' This was in despite of the fact that the university of Montpellier had one of the most renowned medical schools in Europe.[17] In that same year, the French king concluded that the trade of Harfleur had been blighted ' as a result of the wars and the hindrance of our enemies, who have been in the kingdom a long time, burdening and damaging the said port town and its inhabitants, and as a result of the mortality which has been there on several occasions '.[18] Across the Alps in the northern Italian city of Verona, the burden of ' these times of plague and war ' was brought home vividly to the inhabitants in 1438–39. An invasion from Milan and Mantua coincided at that juncture with an attack of plague, and the city governors reported sorrowfully that ' we are battered and dispersed by a combination of war, plague and famine '.[19] Nearer home, the small town of Seaford in Hampshire was reported in1356 as being ' so desolated by plague and the chances of war that men living there are so few and poor that they cannot pay their taxes or defend the town '.[20] This was *conjoncture* in action, and to examine its mechanism is an important goal of the historian.

There are other, more preliminary paths to be trodden, whereby each of the two phenomena can be observed from the inside, but at the same time in relation to one another. The direct effect of plague upon warfare in the later middle ages has been little appreciated. But it is evident that wars could lose some of their impetus as a result of plague, as did the Anglo-French conflict soon after Calais was captured by King Edward III in 1347.[21] The epidemic may also have created problems in recruitment, and in the second half of the fourteenth century men-at-arms had to be offered large financial inducements to serve in the English armies abroad.[22] On a more particular level, campaigns could be hindered by an outbreak of plague, as the Welsh rebel, Owain Glyndŵr, discovered in 1403 ; while he was besieging Caernarvon, ' many of the soldiers been dead there of the pestilence.'[23] The Castilians had a similar experience in 1383 when laying siege to the Portuguese capital, Lisbon : 200 of them expired each day in camp so that eventually more than 2,000 men-at-arms died (aside from archers and others).[24] Armies on the march in difficult country or encamped in inhospitable quarters could be decimated and their fighting capacity much reduced by plague, as John of Gaunt, duke of Lancaster and claimant to the Castilian throne, found to his cost in Castile in 1387, by which date something in the region of two-thirds of his army had been wiped out by the disease.[25]

Equally significant was the effect of warfare upon plague. Like pilgrimages, the movements of armies, embassies and raiding parties could be very effective in spreading the disease both among soldiers and camp-followers and among the civilian population. Equally, the flight of non-combatants from war-torn provinces or from the path of an advancing army might well facilitate the spread of plague elsewhere from an infected community. The interaction of war and disease can be illustrated in the experience of one man, Henry, first duke of Lancaster, who was born at Grosmont in modern Monmouthshire. In 1354 he wrote a highly original treatise called *Le Livre des Seintes Medicines* (Book of Sacred Medicines or Remedies).[26] Its theme, confession of the soul, was common enough in the devotional literature of the age, but as an allegory using medical terminology it is rare indeed. Its vivid pictures of the sick-room, of the bodily afflictions of everyday life, are redolent of Henry's own observations and personal experience. For Henry was renowned as a courteous and chivalrous knight, and he was one of Edward III's most successful commanders in the opening decades of the Hundred Years' War with France. By 1354 he had served on expeditions and in battle many times, particularly in France, and there can be little doubt that the medical lore he recounted in his book was in large part acquired on campaign. The imagery of ' war ' and ' truces ' crops up in the book, and so do wounds, injuries sustained at tournaments, and even the practice of Montpellier's surgeons of dissecting the bodies of criminals for the purpose of instruction. Of plague—or any other specific disease for that matter—there is no direct mention, but it is relevant to note that Henry wrote his book within six years of the plague's outbreak in France and England in 1348, and that he went on expedition to Gascony in 1349 when the epidemic was at its height there. It is ironic that Duke Henry was himself to die in 1361 of plague, during its second major outbreak in the fourteenth century.[27]

Henry of Grosmont is further known to have had several doctors and surgeons in his employ who sometimes accompanied him on his military campaigns. Among them was John Arderne, who has been described as ' the first English surgeon to achieve national fame '.[28] He wrote several medical treatises which went through numerous editions in the late-fourteenth and fifteenth centuries. The practical experience which he emphasised in these writings was probably gained in part when he was abroad with Lancaster in the 1330s and '40s fighting in France, Spain and Flanders. Curiously enough, it was the plague year, 1348-49, which saw his military career as a surgeon end, and his retirement to rural Nottinghamshire begin.

On a more constructive level, war is well acknowledged to be a forcing-ground for medical experiment and the advancement of medical science generally;[29] and what the historian would dearly like to know is the effect that late-mediaeval warfare had on such developments as diagnosis, treatments, operations, and quarantine in relation to the plague that was then rampant. It is striking how valued an element in late-mediaeval armies were the doctors, surgeons and medical trains: at the battle of Agincourt alone in 1415, as many as twenty-four surgeons are known by name to have been present on the English side, carefully organised in medical corps; and the French were no less convinced of the importance of medical officers to their armies.[30] Consider, too, how Richard II's two expeditions to Ireland in the 1390s gave a boost to the trade of English chemists. On both occasions, a surgeon in the king's Household, the famous William Bradewardine, was instructed by the king to buy medicines from the London apothecaries 'for the body of the king and others of his household'. Accordingly, in 1394 Bradewardine bought over £66 worth of medicines, and in 1399 twice as much as that. Unfortunately, there is no indication of what medicines these were or what afflictions they were intended to overcome. Bradewardine, incidentally, had considerable military experience elsewhere, for he was present at the battle of Agincourt and on Henry V's subsequent French compaigns, and he served as constable of Dryslwyn castle in 1399-1402, at the beginning of the Glyndŵr rebellion.[31] Medicine and war were the main theatres of experience in his life.

In this, Bradewardine was not exceptional among contemporary doctors and surgeons. So conscious were some of them of the martial environment in which they practised that they referred to themselves as *miles et physicus* (knight and physician) or *miles in medicinis* (knight in medicine). The military-medical practitioners in the service of the king of Naples did so, and English ones followed suit.[32] The career of Benedetto Regnardati, a doctor from Nursia in central Italy, well illustrates the point. Although he never fought in battle, like others of his family he was employed as a diplomant by the militaristic Italian city states of the fifteenth century. From his medical and diplomatic experiences at a time of incessant internecine warfare and recurrent plague came a treatise entitled *De Preservatione a pestilentia* (On Preservation from the Pestilence) which was written immediately after the 1468 outbreak. He also devised preventive measures to forestall plague in Milan in 1468, and the vision which he had of himself was, to quote his own words, that of *miles et physicus* (knight and physician).[33] Such an impact of war both upon the history of medicine and, more particularly, upon the treatment of plague deserves more attention than it has yet received from historians.

Far more complex and difficult to adduce are the effects of war and plague together on society. Some of them were evidently apparent to contemporaries at places like Vignolles, Montpellier, Harfleur, Verona and Seaford. First and foremost was the depopulation that occurred, not necessarily through death alone but also through the desertion of villages and towns, migration from what was thought to be the vulnerable countryside into the safer town—and *vice versa* in the case of panic-stricken people who fled from town to country. Less easily appreciated by contemporaries themselves, but often detectable in their statements, was the collective psychological depression which was generated by recurrent plague and never-ending campaigning. Thirdly, there was material devastation of property and stock by armies and navies, and the impoverishment of the smaller number of survivors, especially when they were asked to shoulder pre-plague financial burdens. And, finally, in some areas there was a marked inability to defend strategic areas or vulnerable frontiers.[34]

Examples abound of these all too striking effects which, in sum, enable an assessment to be made of the joint impact of war and plague on late-mediaeval society. The family of Richard de la Rivere, a modest Gloucestershire landowner, was badly blighted by death in 1361, most likely by the severe recurrence of plague in that year : his mother Joan died first, and then in September his brother John succumbed ; after burying them both and inheriting their west country property, Richard himself died on 4 December 1361.[35] The death-toll could be just as crippling in war. Michael de la Pole, earl of Suffolk, joined Henry V on his expedition to France in 1415, only to be slain at the battle of Agincourt on 25 October. A month earlier, on 18 September, his eldest son and heir, also named Michael, had died at the siege of Harfleur ; while this Michael's younger brother, William, now earl of Suffolk, had himself to be invalided home from Harfleur and narrowly missed giving death its hat-trick in the de la Pole family.[36]

Yet, as an explanation of depopulation, desertion and flight are recognised as being just as significant as a rocketting death-rate. A Welshman living in Ruthin, Llywelyn ap Madog ap Hywel, ' left his land during the Pestilence on account of poverty '. If Llywelyn was relatively unusual in that in 1354 he ' now came and was admitted by the lord's favour to hold the said land by the service due from the same', his initial impulse to flee was common enough.[37] Witness a Cardiganshire community, plague-ridden and faint-hearted in 1349 : ' there are now only seven and there used to be 104 tenants called *gabularii* who withdrew this year because of the pestilence '.[38]

There was little logical reasoning behind such decisions to flee—certainly no sound medical reasoning. From Messina in Sicily in 1347 ' the population deserted the cities in crowds ; fearing even to stay in the environs, they camped out in the open air in the vineyards '. As Boccaccio noted shortly afterwards of Florence, further north, it was ' as if God in visiting men with this pestilence in requital of their iniquities would not pursue them with His wrath wherever they might be, but intended the destruction of such alone as remained within the circuit of the walls of the city '.[39] By contrast, the town of Albi in southern France apparently reaped considerable benefit in terms of population from plague-induced migration : 492 of the surnames of its inhabitants in 1357 were not present there a mere fourteen years earlier in 1343. The plague of 1348 had supervened.[40] Moreover, the violence associated with warfare was more likely to drive the peasantry into towns than away from them. Paris, whatever population it lost through plague, between 1410 and 1420 served as a haven for country-folk who were anxious to escape the civil strife between the Orlêanist and Burgundian factions.[41]

Nevertheless, when all is said and done, war and plague played a major role in the abandonment of entire communities, and hundreds of so-called ' lost villages ' can be detected in western Europe, many of them ' lost ' or deserted since the demographic crises of the mid-fourteenth century.[42] The county of Northumberland had the third largest number of ' lost ' villages in England, partly because it was a county open to Scottish depredations and border warfare as well as to plague.[43] On the other hand, the village of Tusmore in Oxfordshire was probably deserted as a result of plague alone : by 1358 permission was being granted to turn its fields into a park because every villein there was dead, and even the king's Exchequer was brought to admit that the village no longer had any tax payers.[44]

There were yet other effects that were quite beyond the comprehension of contemporaries, but which historians can attempt to evaluate : the costs of late-mediaeval warfare in monetary, human and material terms, especially during periods of plague and in their aftermath ; the degree of economic contraction in trade, agriculture and industry ; the possibility of economic vitality despite the disruption of war and the blight of plague, as in the arms trade or the slave trade ; the social opportunities open to those who survived illness or benefited from war ; changes in government and politics induced by taxation burdens, monetary inflation, military defeats, or by demands placed on subjects at times of social mobility or social unrest.[45] In all these the conjuncture of war and plague is crucial to an explanation.

Furthermore, there are a number of imponderables which the bacteriologist or the doctor, who is also an historian, can do much to elucidate. While bearing in mind that the symptoms of plague as described by contemporaries were recorded by untrained observers or by people with only rudimentary medical knowledge, the bacteriologist still has useful evidence at his disposal, and there are several questions he can profitably ask of it. In 1970 Professor J. F. D. Shrewsbury produced his massive *A History of Bubonic Plague in the British Isles.* Amid its undoubted virtues lurk several defects.[46] In the first place, it all but ignores the much more lethal septicaemic and pneumonic plagues, both of which are more virulent than the bubonic variety and thrive in rather different climatic and human conditions.[47] There is, therefore, urgent need for a study comparable to Professor Shrewsbury's that is devoted to these two strains of plague. Secondly, Professor Shrewsbury laid some false trails in the investigation of plague in England by too liberally relying on alternative diseases like typhus to explain some of the social disruption of the fourteenth and fifteenth centuries—and especially to explain some of the later plagues after 1348. There is, therefore, a need for a study of several of the other mortal diseases rampant in the middle ages which might have had effects comparable to those of plague—typhus, smallpox and pneumonia spring to mind. Contemporaries, both chroniclers and the writers of medical treatises, were capable of distinguishing most of these diseases from one another and from plague, and it should therefore be possible for the medical historian to do so too.[48] Even more fundamental, perhaps, is another of Shrewsbury's preconceptions —what he describes as the 'invariable' or 'immutable' aetiology of plague, its unchanging character from age to age. A bacteriologist could usefully examine the possibility (to some extent hinted at in relation to nineteenth- and twentieth-century plague) that the aetiology of plague is by no means unchangeable and that the detailed diagnosis of symptoms in the twentieth century need not correspond to those observed in the fourteenth.[49] More investigation needs to be undertaken to establish whether or not plague was a respector of persons or classes in the community. It is undoubtedly true, for example, that most of the plague outbreaks in Paris in the mid-fifteenth century were largely confined to young persons or small children—at least sufficiently so for one observer to comment on it several times.[50] Moreover, although Professor Shrewsbury is at pains to maintain that plague attacks rich and poor alike, there is some evidence that the governing classes of England, both the lay lords and the higher clergy, were more lightly hit than others in the community.[51] An investigation, of the importance of diet, habitation and environment is, therefore, something to which more attention needs to be given. Likewise, the science of immunology might have revealing conclusions to offer: one wonders at the curious immunity which Italian towns in the Alpine foothills enjoyed during the first outbreak of plague in 1348-49, or the city of Milan with its circle of marshes, or Liège with its shielding hills, or the villages of northern England with their poor communications.[52] Important, too, is the personal immunity which a mediaeval man might enjoy during subsequent outbreaks if he managed to survive the first. These are all fields in which direct aid can be sought from the bacteriologist. One final cautionary word needs to be uttered: the medical historian must approach these and other problems initially from the known historical facts, to which medical diagnosis can be applied, rather than by applying to modern principles of diagnosis those historical facts which suit the purpose.

NOTES

1 This paper is substantially as it was delivered at the Congress ; references have been added.

2 For a map of the active, endemic occurrence of plague in the world today, see E. Rodenwaldt (ed.), *World-Atlas of Epidemic Diseases* (3 vols., Falk, Hamburg, 1952-61), Vol. III, map 87.

3 For a map of plague incidence in the mid-fourteenth century, see P. Ziegler, *The Black Death* (Collins, London, 1969), pp. 104-5.

4 E. Perroy, *The Hundred Years War* (London, 1962), provides a general account of the conflict, as well as of civil strife and popular unrest in France.

5 E.g., P. Calvocoressi and G. Wint, *Total War* (Allen Lane, London, 1972), and A. Calder, *The People's War* (Cape, London, 1969), p. 17, quoting Winston Churchill on World War II.

6 C. T. Allmand, 'The War and the Non-combatant', in K. A. Fowler (ed.), *The Hundred Years War* (Macmillan, London, 1971), pp. 163-83 ; *idem, Society at War* (Edinburgh, 1973), ch. V. For 'the people-at-war', see H. J. Hewitt, *The Organisation of War under Edward III* (Manchester University Press, Manchester, 1966), p. vii.

7 *Ibid.*, chs. II-IV ; P. Contamine, *Guerre, État et Société à la fin du Moyen Âge* (Mouton, Paris, 1972) ; C. Singer *et al.* (eds.), *A History of Technology* (5 vols., Clarendon Press, Oxford, 1954-58), Vol. III, ch. 10.

8 E.g., the Black Prince's expedition to Gascony left England in September 1355 and did not return until May 1357 ; the soldiers were recruited as early as May 1355. H. J. Hewitt, *The Black Prince's Expedition of* 1355-1357 (Manchester University Press, Manchester, 1958).

9 Little is known of the plague outbreak in the sixth century, but it appears to have been less widespread than that of the later middle ages. J. Morris, *The Age of Arthur* (Weidenfeld & Nicolson, London, 1973), pp. 222-24 ; W. J. Simpson, *A Treatise on Plague* (University Press, Cambridge, 1905), ch. I.

10 Giovanni Boccaccio, for example, estimated that between March and July 1348 more than 100,000 died within the walls of Florence, a city whose contemporary population has been estimated at about 100,000. Giovanni Boccaccio, *The Decameron:* ed. E. Hutton (Everyman ed., 2 vols., Dent, London, 1930), Vol. I, p. 11 ; G. A. Brucker, *Renaissance Florence* (Wiley, New York, 1969), pp. 25-26, 51, 55 (where plague deaths in 1348 are put at 40,000). At the other extreme, J. F. D. Shrewsbury, *A History of Bubonic Plague in the British Isles* (University Press, Cambridge, 1970), pp. 122-25, arrives at an estimated death-rate in Britain of 5% in 1349.

11 For the plague's recurrence in England, see J. Saltmarsh, 'Plague and Economic Decline in England in the Later Middle Ages', *Camb. hist. J.:* (1941), 7, 23-41 ; J. M. W. Bean, 'Plague, Population and Economic Decline in the Later Middle Ages', *Econ. Hist. Rev.:* (1963), 2 s. 15, 422-37.

12 See Shrewsbury, *Bubonic Plague,* ch. IV (for clerical appointments) ; W. Rees, *South Wales and the March,* 1284-1415 (Oxford U.P.,

London, 1924), pp. 241–52 (for rents) ; K. B. McFarlane, *The Nobility of Later Mediaeval England* (Clarendon Press, Oxford, 1973), pp. 168–71 (for the English nobility and higher clergy) ; D. Herlihy, 'Population, Plague and Social Change in Rural Pistoia, 1201–1430', *Econ. Hist. Rev.*: (1965), 2 s., 18, 225–44 (for tax surveys) ; R. W. Emery, 'The Black Death of 1348 in Perpignan', *Speculum*: (1967), 42, 611–23 (for scribes and lawyers).

13 Contamine, *Guerre, État et Société* ; A. H. Burne, *The Crécy War* (Eyre & Spottiswoode, London, 1955) ; *idem*, *The Agincourt War* (Eyre & Spottiswoode, London, 1956) ; K. B. McFarlane, 'England and the Hundred Years' War', *Past and Present*: (1962), 22, 3–13 ; M. M. Postan, 'The Costs of the Hundred Years' War', *ibid.*: (1964), 27, 34–53, reprinted in M. M. Postan, *Essays on Mediaeval Agriculture and General Problems of the Mediaeval Economy* (University Press, Cambridge, 1973), pp. 63–80 ; and n. 6 above.

14 Hewitt, *Black Prince's Expedition*, ch. II ; H. J. Hewitt, *Cheshire under the Three Edwards* (Chester, 1967), pp. 101–2.

15 *Ibid.*, pp. 95–96.

16 P. S. Lewis, *Later Mediaeval France* (Macmillan, London, 1968), pp. 53, 276.

17 A. M. Campbell, *The Black Death and Men of Learning* (2nd ed., New York, 1966), pp. 151, 147–148.

18 H. A. Miskimin, 'The Last Act of Charles V : the background of the revolts of 1382', *Speculum* : (1963), 38, 434.

19 Archivio di Stato, Verona, Antico Archivio di Comune, Atti del Consiglio, register 58 f. 22r, 33v–34r. I am indebted to Mr. J. E. Law for this reference.

20 Shrewsbury, *Bubonic Plague*, pp. 91–92. See also n. 32 below.

21 Perroy, *Hundred Years War*, pp. 121–24.

22 The growing unpopularity of the French war and increased costs are other explanations. J. W. Sherborne, 'Indentured Retinues and English Expeditions to France, 1369–1380', *English Hist. Rev.* : (1964) 79, 743–44.

23 Rees, *South Wales and the March*, p. 278, n. 6.

24 P. E. Russell, *The English Intervention in Spain and Portugal in the time of Edward III and Richard II* (Clarendon Press, Oxford, 1955), p. 368.

25 *Ibid.*, p. 452.

26 E. J. F. Arnould (ed.), *Le Livre de Seyntz Medicines* (Blackwell, Oxford, 1940) ; *idem*, 'Henry of Lancaster and his "Livre des Seintes Medicines"', *Bull. John Rylands Library* : (1937), 21, 352–86. Until recently only two copies of the treatise were known to exist ; parts of a third have come to light in the National Library of Wales, Aberystwyth. J. Krochalis and R. J. Dean, 'Henry of Lancaster's "Livre de Seyntz Medicines" : new fragments of an Anglo-Norman work', *Nat. Library of Wales Journal* : (1973), 18 (1), 87–94.

27 The most recent study of Duke Henry is K. A. Fowler, *The King's Lieutenant* (Elek, London, 1969).

28 C. H. Talbot and E. A. Hammond, *The Medical Practitioners in Mediaeval England* (Wellcome Historical Medical Library, London, 1965), pp. 111–12.

29 D. Guthrie, *A History of Medicine* (2nd ed., Nelson, London, 1958), ch., XVIII.

30 N. H. Nicolas, *History of the Battle of Agincourt* (repr. of 2nd ed., 1832, Muller, London, 1970), p. 387 ; Talbot and Hammond, *Medical Practitioners, passim ;* Contamine, *Guerre, État et Société,* p. 24.

31 Public Record Office, Exchequer, T. R. ,Council and Privy Seal, 8/657. For Bradewardine, see R. A. Griffiths, *The Principality of Wales in the Later Middle Ages,* Vol. I, *South Wales,* 1277-1536 (University of Wales Press, Cardiff, 1972), pp. 263-64 ; Talbot and Hammond, *Medical Practitioners,* pp. 387-88.

32 *Ibid.*, p. 151 ; J. H. Cotton, ' Benedetto Regnardati of Nursia (1398-1469) ', *Med. Hist.* (1969) 13, 175-76.

33 *Ibid.*, pp. 175-89.

34 Above p. 129. Compare also the financial losses at Newcastle-upon-Tyne by 1350, ' on account of the deadly pestilence as by various other adversities in these times of war ' ; and the plight of Carlisle, which ' is now wasted and more than usually depressed as well by the mortal pestilence lately prevalent in those parts as by frequent attacks ' (by the Scots). Shrewsbury, *Bubonic Plague,* pp. 117, 118.

35 Griffiths, *Principality of Wales,* pp. 110-11.

36 G. E. C.[okayne,] *The Complete Peerage* (12 vols., St. Catherine Press, London, 1910-59), Vol. XII, part 1, 442-43.

37 W. Rees, ' The Black Death in Wales ', *Trans. R. hist. Soc.:* (1920), 4 s. 3, 133, reprinted in R. W. Southern (ed.), *Essays in Mediaeval History* (Macmillan, London, 1968), p. 196.

38 Rees, *South Wales and the March,* p. 244, n.5.

39 F. A. Gasquet, *The Great Pestilence* (Simpkin Marshall, London, 1893), pp. 13, 22 ; Boccaccio, *Decameron,* I, 7-8.

40 G. Prat, ' Albi et la peste noire ', *Annales du Midi:* (1952), 64, 15-25 ; Cf. P. Wolff, *Histoire de Languedoc* (Toulouse, 1967), p. 239.

41 G. Duby, *Rural Economy and Country Life in the Mediaeval West* (Arnold, London, 1968), p. 307.

42 F. Braudel (ed.), *Villages Désertés et Histoire Economique* (Paris, 1965) ; M. Beresford and J. G. Hurst (eds.), *Deserted Mediaeval Villages* (Lutterworth Press, London, 1971).

43 *Ibid.*, pp. 35, 68-69 ; and see also the density map on p. 66.

44 *Ibid.,* p. 8.

45 See, in general, R. H. Bautier, *The Economic Development of Mediaeval Europe* (Thames & Hudson, London, 1971), ch. V.

46 Several of the following criticisms have also been made by C. Morris, ' The Plague in Britain ', *Hist. J. :* (1971), 14, 205-15.

47 L. F. Hirst, *The Conquest of Plague* (Clarendon Press, Oxford, 1953), pp. 27-35.

48 See, for example, the precise contemporary descriptions of symptoms by Guy de Chauliac, Pope Clement VI's physician, in his treatise, ' La Grande Chirurgie ', 1363 (Gasquet, *Great Pestilence,* pp. 43-44) ; and by Nicephorus Gregoras at Constantinople and Geoffrey Le Baker in England (Simpson, *Treatise on Plague*, pp. 21-22, 24-26). See, further, the comments of Morris, *Hist. J. :* (1971), 14, 207-8, 210-11.

49 *Ibid.*, p. 209 ; Shrewsbury, *Bubonic Plague*, p. 110.
50 J. Shirley (ed.), *A Parisian Journal*, 1405-1449 (Clarendon Press, Oxford, 1968), pp. 128, 131, 281.
51 McFarlane, *Nobility of Later Mediaeval England*, pp. 170-71.
52 E.g., Ziegler, *Black Death*, p. 54 ; Shrewsbury, *Bubonic Plague*, p. 1.

PESTIS FLAVA : Y FAD FELEN

John Cule

In the year 1949, in the pages of the *Journal of the History of Medicine*, Sir William MacArthur took issue with Dr J. F. D. Shrewsbury in some detail on the diagnosis of a sixth century plague in the British Isles.[1] The argument was on the nature of the Yellow Plague, known in Welsh as *Y Fad Felen* and in Irish as *Buidhe Connaill.* The forms *Lallwelen* and *Y Dylyt Melen* are also found in Welsh and *Cron Chonnaill* in Irish. All have a common denominator in the later latinisation of *Pestis Flava.* MacArthur's opinion was that it bore all the indications of having been Louse-borne Relapsing Fever due to the *Treponema Recurrentis*—a frequent fellow traveller at the beginnings and ends of Typhus epidemics—and felt that Shrewsbury had made a 'surprising identification of "The Yellow Plague" as confluent Small Pox'. The fact that in the twentieth century, two eminent doctors of medicine felt justified in attempting a specific diagnosis of an obscure pestilence that had occurred some fourteen centuries before is the result of a phenomenon well known to historians. The descriptive detail of an historical event varies in inverse proportion to its proximity in time.

THE RECORD

The first record of any plague that we have in Wales is of the one that brought Saint Brioc, the patron saint of purse makers, in some haste from Brittany to Ceredigion in 526 A.D. The Cardigan parish that now bears his name is Llandyfrïog, within whose confines he perhaps had taken up his abode in answer to the plea.

> The whole Corotician region is overwhelmed
> by a great catastrophe. The inhabitants,
> deprived of thine assistance are mourning ;
> and the one last hope remaining to them of
> escaping so great a peril is, that thou

should'st return to them, and that they may
enjoy thy blessing.[2]

The next record for a pestilence is that of 537 A.D. in the *Annales Cambriae*. The chronicler of the Harleian MS 3859 version adding that it occurred in Ireland as well. But neither of these two early Welsh plagues was characterised as being yellow.

an '	*Gueith camlann inq*ua	year	The grim battle
	arthur & medraut	[537 A.D.]	Camlan in which
	*corrue*runt. et *mortali-*		Arthur and Modred
	[*tas*		fell. and there was
	inbrit-		a mortality
	tannia		in Britain
	et *in hib*er		and in Ireland.
	nia fuit.[3]		

Either could have been the plague that ravaged the year in which Gildas designed his *Lorica* as a charm for his protection against those demons which pestered him.[4]

Gillus hanc loricam fecit ad demones
expellendos eos qui adversaverunt illi
. . . ut non secum trahat me mortalitas huius anni.

The identity of Gildas has exercised many scholars and reminds one of the donnish joke that the *Odyssey* was not written by Homer, but by another man of the same name. The author of the *Lorica* was probably the same Gildas who wrote the historical chronicle *De Excidio Britanniae* with the vituperative *Epistola*. The majority of modern authorities regards these as the work of a single sixth century churchman by the name of Gildas.[5] He himself records his date of birth as the year of the Battle of Badon Hill,[6] now dated at about 500 A.D. And if it is he whose death is recorded in the *Annales Cambriae* for the year 570 A.D., then this plague in his lifetime could have been either that of 526 or 537, or yet again the plague which is the subject of this paper, that of 547 A.D.

In his *Epistola*, Gildas specifically attacks one Magloclunus, amongst the many princes who come in for his castigation, as ' the island dragon . . . sodden with the wine that is pressed from the vine of Sodom '.[7] This refers to Maelgwn Gwynedd, whose death in later accounts is attributed to the Yellow Plague. Gildas found Maelgwn particularly unpleasant, because of his relapse to sinful ways after a period of repentance as a monk. He would have been pleased to have recorded the method and the date on which such a sodomist paid the wages of sin. But in neither the *Lorica* nor in the *Epistola* of his *De Excidio* does he mention that Maelgwn died of the Yellow Plague. This omission could be simply explained if they were all written before 547 A.D., the year in which Maelgwn Gwynedd died.

The third Welsh plague is that of 547 A.D., and like the second is recorded in the *Annales Cambriae.*

an'. Mor-	year.	Great mortality
talitas	[547 A.D.]	in which died Maelgwn
magna		king of north Wales
inqua		
pausat		
mailcun		
rex gene		
dotae.[8]		

The *Annales Cambriae* are amongst the oldest of the Welsh chronicles, recording the happenings between 400 and 977 A.D.[9] The parent MS from which later ones developed was possibly first composed in the late seventh or early eighth century.

The recension of Harleian MS 3859 from which the above two extracts are taken was made in the latter half of the tenth century and contains its copy of the *Annales Cambriae* in an appendage to the *Historia Brittonum* of Nennius. This Welshman of the late eighth and early ninth centuries was a compiler from the works of earlier writers. The world is indebted to him for the story of King Arthur, whose twelve victories are recorded in his chapter 56. The gruesome deaths of princes by poisoning, cut throat, strangling and drowning underline the perils of sovereignty in the Dark Ages and that of Maelgwn results from the plague. Nennius was inventive. He used his ingenuity to defend his countrymen against the sneer of their having no alphabet by promptly inventing a near-Runic one of his own to remedy the deficiency.[10] But he did not, any more than did the *Annales Cambriae* of Harleian MS 3859, paint the plague of Maelgwn with any particular colour.

Geoffrey of Monmouth was not the man to miss a little embellishment to help a story along, but even he does not appear to have been responsible for the gilding of the plague of 547 A.D. He wrote during the literary revival of the twelfth century, in which he claims his place as a literary historian, a different breed from the chronicler. Geoffrey was the populariser of the Arthurian legend and his work is based on such sources as Gildas, Nennius and Bede, *plus* the inventive genius of Geoffrey. Some 200 manuscripts of his history are known, with 6 independent Welsh translations as the bases of 50 surviving manuscripts composed between the thirteenth and sixteenth centuries.[11] His work was so notoriously unreliable that Giraldus Cambrensis recorded the story of the Welshman possessed by evil spirits, who was relieved when the Gospel according to Saint John was placed upon his bosom. When Geoffrey's book was substituted, as a sort of therapeutic test, the spirits settled not only upon his body, but even upon the book itself, both in greater numbers and for a longer time than usual.[12]

A late fourteenth or early fifteenth century Welsh version of Geoffrey's History, *Ystorya Brenhined Y Britanyeit* of the *Red book of Hergest* says this of Maelgwn Gwynedd.

> *Ac yn eglwys ger llaw degannwy*
> *yny gastell ehun ybu varw.*[13]
>
> And in the church nearby Deganwy
> within his own castle he died.

It will be seen that in this late Welsh copy of Geoffrey's *History*, the Welsh copyist merely stated the fact of death and did not add any further detail, although the term yellow plague had already appeared in the two thirteenth century manuscripts quoted below. Although, of course, he was not necessarily aware of them. The first of these could have been found in a manuscript of the *Annales Cambriae,* written in an abridged copy of the Domesday Book, probably compiled in 1286 A.D., the date of the last entry. The bracketed portions of the extract below distinguish the later additions of this manuscript.

> CIII *Annus. Mortalitas magna*
> (*fuit in Britannia*) *in qua pausat*
> *Mailcun rex Genedotae.* (*Unde dicitur,*
> '*Hir hun Mailgun en llis Ros*'. *Tunc*
> *fuit lallwelen*).[14]

[547 A.D.]
CIII Year. There was a great mortality (in Britain) in which
Maelgwn king of north Wales died. (Thence it is said,
' The long sleep of Maelgwn in the Court of Rhos '. Then
there was a yellow plague).

Thus it came about that it was some seven hundred years after the pestilence that a written record of its yellowness is noted in any extant record of the *Annales Cambriae.* But it is not the earliest record of the Yellow Plague. There had been earlier although somewhat less reliable additions of this detail by two literary historians. The biographer of the Life of Saint Teilo not only added the detail but enlarged on it with a few clinical and therapeutic observations.

It was called the Yellow Pestilence,
because it occasioned all people who were seized by it,
to be yellow and without blood . . .
If anyone endeavoured to apply a remedy to the sick person
not only had the medicines no effect,
but the dreadful disorder brought the physician,
together with the sick person, to death.
For it seized Maelgwn, King of North Wales,
and destroyed his country.[15]

It is interesting that the name of the epidemic is twice given in Welsh ; first as *lallwellen* in an otherwise Latin text of the *Breviate of Domesday Book* and again in Welsh as *Y Dylyt Melen* in the Latin text of the ' Life of Saint Oudoceous '. Is there a clue here to a missing and yet earlier common source of Welsh origin ?

Dr Wendy Davies believes that the charters of the *Book of Llandaff,* in which book the Life of Saint Teilo appears, were edited in the early twelfth centry.[16] Morgan Watkin, on linguistic grounds believes the work to date from the early thirteenth century.[17] Not all historians have been happy about its reliability. R. Ian Jack referred to the *Book of Llandaff* as ' The oldest and most notorious of Welsh ecclesiastical compilations ' ; E. D. Jones remarked that it was ' to be used with caution ' ; and Christopher Brooke commented that it ' could have been written by Geoffrey of Monmouth himself '.[16]

Saint Teilo, also known as Eliud, was born in Penally in south Pembrokeshire. He was a disciple of Saint Dubricius, studied with

Paulinus at Llanddeusant, north Carmarthenshire and became associated with Saint David. It was said that following the pilgrimage of saints David, Padarn and Teilo to Jerusalem, Teilo had to flee to Brittany following his return home to Wales in order to avoid the Yellow Plague and chanced to meet his nephew Saint Oudoceous in the course of his flight. The Yellow Plague was likened to ' a column of a watery cloud ' sweeping over the ground as a shower of rain sweeps along low lying valleys.[15] It bears an interesting resemblance to a description in Adomnan's *Life of Saint Columba* (d.597) of a rain cloud which would drop pestiferous rain on Ireland, giving rise to festering sores on human bodies and the udders of animals. A description that can give rise to speculations of Cow Pox !

> Men and cattle who suffer from them,
> afflicted with that poisonous disease, will
> be sick even unto death.[18]

The other literary historian of the twelfth - thirteenth centuries who refers to the *Pestis Flava* in the time of Saint Tei lo is Giraldus Cambrensis (1146-1223) writing in his *De Invectionibus;*

> *quam flavam pestem vocabant, quam et physici*
> *ictericium dicunt passionem.*[19]

The people call it the Yellow Plague, but the physicians know the disease as icterus, a nicety of distinction in professional terminology. In all probability, this is the earliest of our twelfth-thirteenth century examples and thus the first known record in which the term yellow is applied to the sixth century plague, and a good six centuries later. Did however, Giraldus and the compilers of the *Book of Llandaff*, as well as the copyist of the *Annales* on the fly leaves of the *Breviate of Domesday Book*, have a common source that is now lost ? Did Geoffrey of Monmouth miss it too, or if such a document existed was it made after his time ?

Before moving on to the final act with the full flowering of the epidemiology, one should turn, if only briefly, to the Irish sources on which MacArthur based much of his evidence.

It has already been noted above that the Harleian MS recension of the *Annales Cambriae* mentions that the plague of 537 also took place in Ireland. There is nothing in the Welsh evidence to make this the year of *Y Fad Felen,* which is associated with the plague of 547, the year in which Maelgwn Gwynedd died. It therefore becomes necessary to compare the Irish Annals of this period. MacArthur has argued at some length on his reasons for believing that *buidhe conail,* the yellow plague or *crom connaille,* the saffron plague was due to the Relapsing Fever.[1]

The evidence of the *Annals of Tigernach* in Bodleian MS Rawlinson B488 is a section written in the thirteenth century containing in unglossed form a reference to the *mortalitas magna* of 550 A.D. including the Irish words *Crom Conaille* and *buidhe conail.*[20]

Editors introduce new hazards. O'Conor in his edition of the *Annals of Tigernach,* under A.C. 550, introduces in his Latin translation the confusing term *flava scabies* for *Crom Conaill,* although this does not occur in the original.[21] The thirteenth century recension of the *Annals of Tigernach* refer to the yellow or saffron plague. The entry for A.D. 543 identifies the *mortalitas magna* of that year as *Blefed,* the name by which the Irish annalists refer to Bubonic Plague.[22]

The *Annals of Boyle* record in 534 A.D. a great mortality to which a glossator, in a hand not much later than the thirteenth century one of the text has added *buidhe chonaill.*[23] The Irish annalists appear to have distinguished *blefed* and *crom conaille* at some period in or possibly earlier than the thirteenth century.

The spread of Plague in Europe and Asia at about this period may be studied from other sources. Procopius, the Greek historian gives an unmistakeable account of the outbreak of Bubonic Plague at Constantinople, which in its spread included the emperor Justinian, ' for he too had a swelling of the groin '.[24] This epidemic is believed to have started in Egypt and by 543 A.D. had spread to France,[25] for Gregory of Tours states the groin pestilence broke out eight years before Saint Gall's death, which occurred in 551 A.D.[26] A plague is recorded in Britain and Ireland about this time, but unfortunately diagnostically significant references to swellings in the groin are absent. Likewise in Europe references to a yellow plague are absent. The reasons for their absence may be that the manuscripts are lost, but this supposition can scarcely be adduced as evidence for a diagnosis. For an epidemic characterised as yellow, MacArthur makes a convincing case for an identification as Relapsing Fever. Relapsing Fever is frequently seen in association with that other famine fever, Typhus. Bubonic plague was recorded in Europe. It is possible that all three occurred coincidentally, or in close succession, to make a confusing picture for a contemporary lay chronicler, an impossible differential diagnosis for a contemporary physician but an interesting academic exercise for later medical historians. But these last must first carefully consider all the evidence. Were these early records of yellow plague culled from parent MSS now lost ? Or were they in themselves the beginnings of the undoubted legendary additions which now follow ?

THE LEGEND

The antiquarians and literary historians of the nineteenth century were given to imaginative reconstructions, often of considerable charm, which must be used with great caution by those whose concern with history is to learn what really happened. The literary skills of Lady Charlotte Guest, to whom the Welsh are indebted for her translation of the *Mabinogion*, must bear some of the responsibility for the spread of the romantic version of the Yellow Plague. The note of caution is sounded for the historian when he learns that her adviser was Mr T. Williams, the son of the man who outshone Geoffrey of Monmouth for his invention, Iolo Morganwg.

It becomes apparent that the romantic story of the quarrel of the bard Taliesin with Maelgwn Gwynedd, related by Lady Charlotte Guest as *Hanes Taliesin* at the end of her classic translation of the Mabinogion, is based on accounts of the legend derived from Iolo. In this she was advised by his son and consulted the latter's edition of the *Iolo MSS*.[27]

The tale she tells is how Elphin, Taliesin's master, and one of the many princes sacrificed to Maelgwn's pride was imprisoned for his imprudent double boast of the virtue of his wife and the skill of his bard ; there being some suggestion that both were of a better quality than those of Maelgwn. Taliesin by a combination of skill and magic was fortunately able to confound the tyrant and furthermore deliver his master from the prison of thirteen locks into which he had been cast. In the last stage of the competition finals in which he won supremacy over the king's bards he is heard to prophesy.

Be silent, then, ye unlucky rhyming bards,
For you cannot judge between truth and falsehood.
If you be primary bards formed by heaven,
Tell your king what his fate will be.
It is I who am a diviner and a leading bard,
And know every passage in the country of your king ;

I shall liberate Elphin from the belly of the stony tower ;
And will tell your king what will befall him.
A most strange creature will come from the sea marsh of Rhianedd
As a punishment of iniquity on Maelgwn Gwynedd ;
His hair, his teeth, and his eyes being as gold,
And this will bring destruction upon Maelgwn Gwynedd.[28]

The symbolism of the monster in relation to the yellow plague seems tailor made and when her source of the poem is disclosed, it does appear that Lady Charlotte Guest has accepted Iolo Morganwg's attribution of it to Taliesin.[29]

Not enough was known in Lady Charlotte's day for her to have been able to distinguish between the historical sixth century Taliesin, a bard who lived in what is now south west Scotland, and that legendary figure of Taliesin who emerged in the ninth century. Whilst there is authentic work which may be attributed to the historical poet found in part of *Llyfr Taliesin* or *The Book of Taliesin*, there is also *Hanes Taliesin* or *The Story of Taliesin*, which recounts the doings of the legendary figure of the *Chwedl Taliesin* or *Legend of Taliesin.* Confusion would be worse confounded if Iolo had a hand in what was already a mixture of truth and tale for centuries before his time.

Lady Charlotte Guest had made her translation of Taliesin's prophecy from the *Myvyrian Archaiology* of Iolo, wherein appears a variant of a poem known as *Dymma Fustl y Beirdd.* After the ending of this poem as accepted by the ' learned Mr John Jones of Gelli Lyfdu ' one finds the romantic passage above as transcribed and then translated by Lady Charlotte.[30]

The chilly thought of a search for Iolo's sources, all too likely to prove at best of doubtful provenance seemed the next and necessary step. Fortunately, in the event it proved unnecessary, because Mr Gerallt Harries, who was aware of my problem, most generously shared with me the good fortune of his discovery of an earlier version. It occurs in a text of *Chwedl Taliesin* in BM Add MS 31055 and was ascribed by its copyist and editor, none other than the erudite physician and lexicographer, Syr Tomas Wiliems (1545-?1622) to the sixth century bard.[31] This attribution has not been accepted by modern scholarship.

Lady Charlotte Guest then also gave publicity in her enormously popular translation of the *Mabinogion* to the following confidently expressed account of the death of Maelgwn Gwynedd.

> He died of the Vad Velen, or Yellow Pestilence usually called the Yellow Plague of Rhos, which was said to have been caused by the number of unburied bodies of the slain that remained on that spot, and whoever went within reach of the effluvia fell dead immediately.
> To avoid the effects of this pestilence it is said that Maelgwn retired from his castle of Dyganwy, to the church of Llanrhos, where he hoped to remain, shut up in the sanctuary, safe from all danger ; but being impelled by curiosity, he looked out through the keyhole of the door, and thereby caught the infection, thus fulfilling the prediction uttered by Taliesin— . . .
> This plague lasted from the year 557 to 562, and its ravages were fearful in the extreme. A Triad records it as one of the three direful maladies, and is even employed as an image of horror in the compositions of the Bards.[32]

The first and the last paragraphs of this tale come straight from Iolo Morganwg's spurious triads, *Trioedd Ynys Prydain.*[33] The middle paragraph could well have derived from the *Iolo MSS*, edited by the son on whom Lady Charlotte relied wherein is this passage, attributed to a sixteenth century MS of Sion Cent (1367?-1430?)

> *. . . a Maelgwn Gwynedd a'i gweles drwy dwll y clo yn Eglwys Rhos, ag a fu farw o'i gweled.*
>
> . . . And Maelgwn Gwynedd beheld the Yellow Plague through the keyhole in the church door and forthwith died.[34]

Again I am indebted to Mr Gerallt Harries for a further discovery of his in the hand of Robert Vaughan of Hengwrt (?1592-1667) and ante-dating at least Iolo Morganwg, if not Sion Cent.

> *Maelgwn a fu farw wedi gweled y Vad Velen drwy dwll ar ddor yr eglwys lle i raethau i ymgadw rhag eu gweled hi.*
>
> *hen lyfr*

Maelgwn died after seeing the Fad Felen through
a hole in the door of the church to which he had
gone to protect himself from seeing it.
old book.[35]

Thomas Love Peacock made yet more of the story in his *Misfortunes of Elphin,* of which the Gregynog Press made such a fine edition.[36]

From whence came these accounts that an historian of the twentieth century can write of the 'yellow plague which swept across Europe' and medical historians discuss its epidemiology ?[37] The only evidence available at present seems to be limited to Wales and Ireland and written half a millenium later, and for which a convincing source has yet to be found.

REFERENCES AND NOTES

1 MacArthur, W., 'Comments on Shrewsbury's "The Yellow Plague"', *J. Hist. Med.,* (1950, 5, 214-215.) also 'Famine Fevers in England and Ireland', *J. Br. Archaeol. Ass.,* (1944), 3, s., 9, 66–71.
Shrewsbury, J. F. D., *J. Hist. Med.,* (1949), 4, 5-47.

2 Doble, G. H., *Saint Brioc,* 'Cornish Saints' Series No. 17, Reprinted from *Pax,* 1928, s.41.
The passage is taken from Doble's translation of the *Vita Brioccii* found at Rouen. The *Vita* was printed by Dom Plaine in 1883 and dated by him, on calligraphical evidence, as belonging to the 11th or 12th centuries. The original MS was believed to have been written before 850 A.D. by an unknown biographer. *Analecta Bollandiana* (1883), 2, 161-190, and supplement in *Analecta* (1904), 23, 264-265.

3 Phillimore, E., 'The *Annales Cambriae* and Old Welsh Genealogies from Harleian MS 3859', *Y Cymmrodor,* (1888), 9, 154.

4 Williams, H., (ed.) *Gildae de Excidio Britanniae, fragmenta, liber de paenitentia, accedit et Lorica Gildae,* Hon. Soc. Cymmrodorion, London, 1899, p. 304. (From *The Lorica*).
Singer, Charles, *From Magic to Science,* Dover Publications, New York, 1958. p. 119.
(See this work for Singer's essay, 'The Lorica of Gildas the Briton. A magical text of the sixth century').

5 Jack, R. Ian, *Medieval Wales:* (The Sources of History : Studies in the use of Historical Evidence) Hodder & Stoughton, London, 1972. pp. 15-19.

6 Williams, H., *op. cit.,* pp. 60–62.

7 Williams, H., *op. cit., p.* 77. (From *De Excidio*).

8 Phillimore, E., *op. cit.*, p. 155. (From Harleian MS 3859).
9 Jones, Thomas, *Brut y Tywysogyon or The Chronicle of the Princes*, (Peniarth MS 20 Version), University of Wales Press, Cardiff, 1952, see pp. xl,
10 Jack, R. Ian, *op. cit.*, p. 20.
11 Jack, R. Ian, *op. cit.*, pp. 26–29.
12 Gerald of Wales; Giraldus de Barri, *The Itinerary of Archbishop Baldwin through Wales, A.D. MCLXXXVIII*, (tr. by Sir Richard Colt Hoare), Vol. 1, William Miller, London, 1806, p. 106. (From Book 1, Chapter V, *Itinerarium Cambriae*).
13 Rhys, J. & Evans, J. G. (eds.) The *Text of the Bruts from the Red Book of Hergest*, Clarendon Press, Oxford, 1890. p. 234. (From '*Ystorya Brenhined y Brytanyeit*': a Welsh Version of Geoffrey of Monmouth's *Historia Regum* Britanniae.)
14 Ab Ithel, Rev. John Williams, (ed.) *Annales Cambriae*, Rolls Series XX, Longman, London, 1860, p. 4.
15 Rees, W. J., *The Liber Landavensis*, William Rees for the Welsh MSS Society, Llandovery, 1840., pp. 343–4 (p. 101 of Latin text). (From the 'Life of St. Teilo'.) There is a similar account of the Yellow Plague in the Life of St. Oudoceous. (*ibid*, p. 371) (pp. 123–4 of Latin text). '. . . after a very long time, the Yellow Pestilence came to the Greater Britain, which was called Yellow, because it occasioned all persons who were seized by it, to be yellow and very pallid . . .'
16 Jack, R. Ian, *op. cit.*, pp. 143–5.
17 Watkin, M., 'The Chronology of the Annales Cambriae and the Liber Landavensis on the basis of their old French Graphical Phenomena'. *Natn. Lib. Wales J.* (Summer 1960), 11 (3), 181–226.
18 Anderson, A.O. & M.O. (eds.) *Adomnan's Life of Columba*, Nelson, London, 1961, pp. 331–3.
19 Brewer, J.S., (ed.) *Giraldi Cambrensis Opera*, Rolls Series, XXI, Vol. III, Longman, London, 1863, p. 151. (From De Jure et Statu Menevensis Ecclesiae.)
20 Bodleian MS Rawlinson B 488, fol. 8 recto, col. a, lines 11–12.
21 O'Conor, C. (ed.), *Rerum Hibernicarum Scriptores Veteres*, Tom II, T. Payne, London, 1825. p. 139.
22 Bodleian MS Rawlinson B 488. Entry for A.D. 543. *Kal. Jan. fer.* 1, *anno postquam Papa Vigilius obiit, Mortalitas magna que* Blefed *dicitur, in qua* Mobi Clarinach, *cui nomen est* Berchan, *obiit.* (From O'Donovan, J., *Annals of the Kingdom of Ireland by the Four Masters . . .*, 2nd ed., Dublin, 1856, Vol. 1, fn. p. 183.)
23 British Museum MS Cotton Titus A xxv, f. 14b. I am indebted to T. C. Skeat, Keeper of Manuscripts for this information.
24 Procopius of Caesarea, *History of the Wars*, Book II, xxiii, 20, (H. B. Dewing's translation, Loeb Classics, Heinemann, London, 1914, Vol. 1, p. 473.)
25 Gregory of Tours, *The History of the Franks*, Book IV, Chapter 5. (O. M. Dalton's translation Clarendon Press, Oxford, 1927, Vol. II, p. 119).
26 MacArthur, W. P., 'The identification of some pestilences recorded in

the Irish annals', *Irish Hist. Stud.*, (March 1949), 6 (23), fn 6, p. 173 (pp. 169-188).

27 Williams, T., (ab Iolo), *Iolo MSS*, William Rees for the Welsh MSS Society, Llandovery, 1848, pp. 460-1, 466-7.

28 Guest, Lady Charlotte, *The Mabinogion*, Longman, London and Rees, Llandovery, 1849, Vol. 3, p. 377. (Welsh transcription on p. 343 'supplied from The Myvyrian Archaiology, Vol. I. pp. 20 and 26'. This was the first edition, S. Rousseau, London, 1801.)

Another romantic version of Maelgwn and Taliesin is given by Thomas Love Peacock in *The Misfortunes of Elphin*, The Gregynog Press, 1928.

29 Guest, Lady Charlotte, *op. cit.*, pp. 390-6 (From '*Notes to Taliesin*').

30 Jones, O., Williams, E. & Pughe, W. O., (eds.) *The Myvyrian Archaiology of Wales, collected out of Ancient MSS*, 2nd ed., Thomas Gee, Denbigh, 1870, pp. 29 & 35. Lady Charlotte used the 1st ed. Cf ref. 28.

31 BM add MS 31055, fol. 133v. (I am indebted to Mr Gerallt Harries for his help with this reference and note). *Bustl y Beirdd* is a poem which belongs clearly to *Chwedl Taliesin*. It does not occur in the *Book of Taliesin*, but occurs frequently in MSS from the first half of the 16th century onwards. (At least 47 copies of it are known.) The earliest extant one is probably that in Cardiff MS 5, p. 104, written in 1527 by Elis Gruffudd. The copy which Sir Ifor Williams quotes in his *Canu Taliesin* is that which John Jones of Gellilyfdy wrote into his Peniarth MS 111 about 1610. John Jones has included two copies of the poem in this MS, at pages 284-5 and 366-8. The first copy ends thus :-
Taliesin ai gwnaeth yn llys Maelgwn Gwynedd o lid wrth y glêr. (*Clêr*=poets).

The second copy, on pp. 366-8 contains four additional lines (which are also found in the Cardiff MS 5 recension as well as in other copies of the poem).

Following *Bustl y Beirdd* on pp. 368-9 of Peniarth MS 111 John Jones wrote a brief prefatory note to a short additional poem, explaining that it may perhaps not be the work of Taliesin. In fact he leaves a blank at the end, omitting to give its author a name. He furthermore states that he is in some doubt from his examples, whether there should be a break in the text here. This poem is a variant of Taliesin's prophecy.

Tewch chwi, bosfeirdd ffeilstion anhylwydd;
Mi wyddoch chwi rannu rhwng gwir a chelwydd;
Myfi y sydd ddewin a phrifardd cyffredin
A edwyn bob orsin yng nghyrre'r Gorllewin;
O rhyddhaf i Elffin o vol y tŵr meinin,
Mi a fynaga i'r brenin gwbwl o'i gyfrin.

Ef a ddaw pryf rhyfedd i forfa y rhianedd;
Ei flew fydd eurwedd, ei lygaid a'i ddannedd;
A hwnnw a wna ddiwedd am Faelgwn Gwynedd.

There is a copy written by Syr Tomas Wiliems, the great lexicographer, which is probably earlier, and may well be the earliest extant copy of the above short poem. It occurs in his hand in B.M. Add. MS 31055, fol. 133v., where it follows his copy of the poem *Dyhuddiant Elffin* (also a part of *Chwedl Taliesin*) rather than *Bustl y Beirdd*. It is interesting to note that Syr Tomas does attribute this poem to Taliesin, and does not share John Jones's doubts. He omits the first two lines of John Jones's copy, and as his copy has so many variants it is included here :-

Myfi sydd ddewin a phrifardd Cyffredin:
Ac adwaen bob gorsin yng ngogof Gorllewin ;
Mi a ryddhaf Elffin o fol y tŵr meinin ;
Mi a fynagaf i'ch brenin ac i'r holl gyffredin.

E ddaw pryf rhyfedd i Forfa Rhianedd
I ddial enwiredd ar Faelgwyn Gwynedd ;
A'i flew a'i ddannedd a'i lygaid yn euredd ;
A hwn a wna ddiwedd ar Faelgwyn Gwynedd.
Taliesin

There are later copies in Mostyn MS 163, p. 228. B.M. Add. MS 14867, p. 58 ; B.M. Add. MS 15002, p. 65 and Panton MS 14, i, 148. The *Reports on Welsh MSS* (HMSO) note that the copy of *Bustl y Beirdd* in Cardiff MS 67 ends with the last line of the above short poem, so that this poem is presumably added on to *Bustl y Beirdd* in that MS which was written about 1695. The earlier copies treat them as separate poems.

32 Guest, Lady Charlotte, *op. cit.*, pp. 399-400.

33 Jones, Williams & Pughe, *op. cit.*, p. 401.

34 Williams, T. (ab Iolo), *op. cit.*, p. 78.

35 National Library of Wales MS 9094 A, folio 83 recto. (I am indebted to Mr Gerallt Harries for this reference and his transcript from it below of the notes on Maelgwn Gwynedd in the hand of Robert Vaughan of Hengwrt (1592?-1667) and probably written between 1650 and 1660).

hûn hir Vaelgwn yn Eglwys Rôs
Dihareb

Maelgwn a fu farw wedi gweled y Vad
Velen drwy dwll ar ddor yr eglwys
lle i raethau i ymgadw rhag eu gweled hi.
hen lyfr

Tri lleithigllwyth y.p. [*ynys prydain*] *Arthur yn pen teyrnedd ynghaer lleon ar wysg, Dewi yn pen esgys a Maelgwn G : yn pen hyneif.*
Trioedd

Tempore Ida Nordorum regis floruit Taliesinus et Malcunus magnus apud Britones in regione Guenedotiae regnavit.

Nennius

Whilst Saint Patern was bishop of Mauritania yt is to say llan Patern vawr. Mailgun king of North Wales came wth an armie to to [sic] subdue South Wales.

Io : Tinmuth

An^{0}. 540 *Paternus postquam pro annos.* 21. *in llanpaternensi ecclesia vixisset in Armoricam revocatus ventensem epantum isi octavit.*
heare by it appeares yt Mailgwn was king of Northwales before 540, wch the Triades before menconed doth confirme when it intimateth ye king.

Arthur & Mailgwn & St D*avi*d Flourished in the same time. And therefore it is most probable yt Maelgwn flourished in king Idas tyme. who began to raigne. A^{0}. 547 and ruled 12 yeares yt is to a^{0}. 559 as Nenni*us* signifieth.

Malgwn died of ye iaundizo (*Wedi gweled y Vâd felen*). *Ictericia pestis ille Mailcono in Guenedocia regnante erupisse dicitur. Liber Landaff.* to know when this plague happened consider yt St Samson was bishop of Dôl in little Britayne [Britanny] when Teilaw for feare of that plague came to little Britaine wth Samson certainly flourished *temporibus Childeberti regis. vsque :* 75. who began his raigne a^{0} 515 & died a^{0} 560.

36 Peacock, Thomas Love, *The Misfortunes of Elphin,* The Gregynog Press, 1928.

37 Williams, A.H., *An Introduction to the History of Wales,* University of Wales Press Board, Cardiff, 1969, p. 75.

MEDDYGON MYDDFAI

Howard E. F. Davies and Morfydd E. Owen

The traditions which have grown up around Meddygon Myddfai, or the Physicians of Myddfai, a small village in north Carmarthenshire, are a good example of how threads of folklore, popular traditions and learned writings can become fused together in the memory of a people. The folk-tale of Llyn y Fan Fach in the Carmarthenshire Van identifies the descendants of a union between a lake fairy and a mortal with a line of hereditary country doctors.[1] This folk-tale has diverted attention somewhat from the few facts available about Meddygon Myddfai and the nature of the collections of medical writings associated with their name in the Welsh literary tradition.

Our purpose in this twenty-minute paper is to ignore the fairy tale and to discuss the evidence for the history of the family of Myddfai and the medieval medical texts connected with their name.

From the XIVth century on, the fame of Meddygon Myddfai is attested in popular Welsh literary and oral tradition. Families possessing certain medical knowledge and skills are recorded as holding lands in the Carmarthenshire parish of Myddfai, farms and holdings like Llwyn Ifan Feddyg and Llwyn Maredudd Feddyg.[2] A certain south-facing slope on Mynydd Myddfai, rich in ferns, bog plants and lichens is called Pant y Meddygon, and here traditionally the doctors collected the plants and herbs for their remedies. The last of the line of hereditary physicians recorded as having practised at Myddfai were two XVIIIth century figures, father and son, whose grave is at the church and whose deaths are recorded in the Parish Register—one David Jones, *chirurgor,* who died in 1719, and John Jones, his son, who died in 1739.[3]

Lewis Morris, the XVIIIth century antiquary, is reputed to have met the son of the latter, who had abandoned the calling either 'because he considered it beneath him or because he was brought up to other things'.[4] Distant descendants of the family continued to practise medicine until this century. The *Welsh Medical Gazette* lately published photographs of two recent members.[5] This then is the popular tradition. The learned tradition is derived from the fact that associated with this family are certain medieval writings preserved in manuscripts. Some of these belong to the XIVth century, other are later copies. These medical writings are prefixed by one or two introductory passages or colophons.

COLOPHON I

Here with the help of God, the Almighty Lord, are shown the most important and essential remedies for man's body. And those who caused them to be written down in this manner were Rhiwallon the doctor and his sons, Cadwgan, Gruffudd and Einion : for they were the best and leading doctors of their time and the time of Rhys Gryg, their lord and Lord of Dinefwr, the man who safeguarded their status and privilege completely and honourably as was their due. And the reason they caused the rules of their art to be written down in this way was lest there be no one who knew them as well as they did after their days.

COLOPHON II

This book was put together from the various books of the physicians and doctors, such books as have been proved to be correct, namely the books of Rhiwallon the doctor, and his sons, namely Cadwgan, Gruffudd and Einion.

Every doctor should know these rules and keep them well, lest his art fail him, and the patient is blinded or some such thing, because of his error or lack of knowledge.

The first colophon suggests that Rhiwallon and his sons came into prominence under the patronage of Rhys Gryg, Lord of Dinefwr, and that they possessed certain basic medical skills and knowledge which they committed to writing in the vernacular. The second colophon suggests that the writings of Rhiwallon had gained a certain reputation and were used as source books by other doctors, or conversely, in the manner of the Middle Ages, the fame of the family was such that it added authenticity and weight to the value of any fresh medical text to attribute it to their authorship.

We should like first to examine the plausibility of the historical references in the first Colophon. Rhys Gryg[6] (or Rhys the Stammerer, or Rhys the Small) who died in 1233 was one of the eight sons of Rhys ap Gruffudd ap Rhys, or the Lord Rhys who died in 1197, one of the most important of the last native Welsh princes. The family of the Lord Rhys is known not only for political achievements but also for patronage of the church, the arts and of learning. He and his descendants were known as patrons of the Cistercian Abbeys of Whitland and Strata Florida, great centres of native learning. The Lord Rhys founded the Premonstratensian Abbey of Tal-y-Llychau. Some of the recensions of the Welsh law texts, the Welsh Chronicles, *Brut y Tywysogion,* and the Latin *Chronica de Wallia*, the translations of certain religious texts were among the works which seem to have been sponsored by the family. They were thus well-known patrons of learning—both Latin and vernacular. It would not be unlikely that such a line should support the learning of a family of medical men, particularly at a time when medical studies were gaining prominence in Europe generally.

The Lord Rhys had amassed for himself a substantial Lordship.[7] His sons, at his death, succeeded to portions of it. The heart of the Deheubarth regime of the Lord Rhys were the two *cantrefi* (or Hundreds) of Cantref Mawr and Cantref Bychan, containing the *caput* of the whole domain Dinefwr and the old ecclesiastical capital at Llandeilo Fawr. After his father's death, these *cantrefi* passed into the hands of Rhys Gryg. The *cantrefi* of Medieval Wales were divided into administrative units or *cymydau* of which there were three in Cantref Bychan, Iscennen, Perfedd and Hirfryn, the *cymydau* into economic units or *maenorau,* consisting of groups of bond or free villes or *trefi*. During the XIIIth century, Myddfai was a royal manor inhabited by freemen directly under the lordship of Dinefwr, and for much of his rule under the lordship of Rhys Gryg, who held Dinefwr almost continuously from 1222-1233, and who is referred to by the poets as '*llyw Dinefwr*'.[8] That is, Myddfai was a manor where the lord might well settle some of his court officials. Dr John Cule has shown how the Welsh laws,

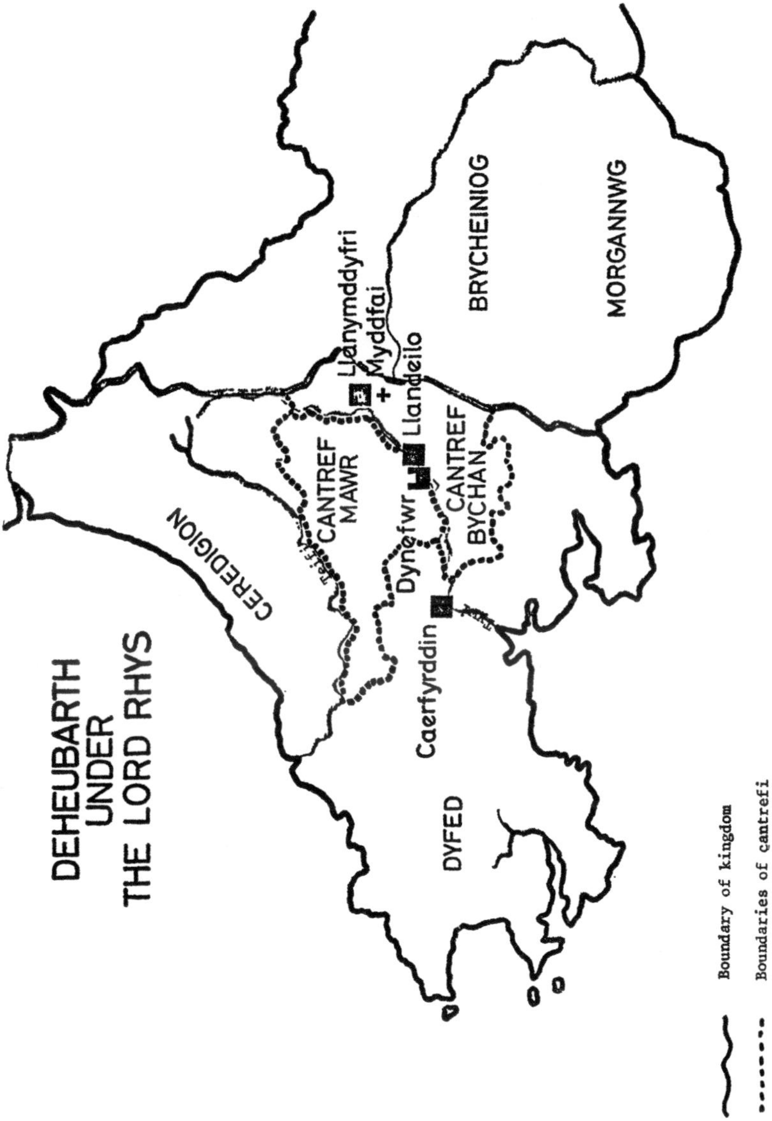
DEHEUBARTH
UNDER
THE LORD RHYS
CEREDIGION
CANTREF
MAWR
CANTREF
BYCHAN
Llanymddyfri
Myddfai
Llandeilo
Dynefwr
Caerfyrddin
BRYCHEINIOG
MORGANNWG
DYFED
Boundary of kingdom
Boundaries of cantrefi

the earliest surviving recensions of which stem from the period of Rhys Gryg, describe the privileges of the royal mediciner among the officials of the Welsh courts.[9] He was a layman and was reputed to possess a free franchise. Myddfai was a manor of free tenants. By the end of the XIIIth century all Wales had fallen to the Anglo-Normans. The *cymydau* of Hirfryn and Perfedd in Cantref Bychan became part of the Lordship of Llanymddyfri. Surveys of this lordship record a most unusual due of service, namely that the ten free tenants of the Maenor of Myddfai were obliged to furnish the Lord of Llanymddyfri with a doctor to follow him on his progress throughout Wales.[10]

The great marcher lords of the XIIIth and XIVth centuries inherited a social structure and pattern of regalia from the native rulers which they did their best to maintain, particularly, when the regalia were advantageous to them.[11] It seems possible, in view of the colophon, and the evidence of the survey, that lands in Myddfai were held by a family of lay physicians originally mediciners of the Lords of Dinefwr and subsequently of the Anglo-Norman Lords of Cantref Bychan and finally, if popular tradition may be accepted, a family of country physicians famous for their remedies and their books.

Such a story is not without its parallels in Celtic societies. One of the features of early Celtic society in Ireland, Scotland and Wales was the emergence, in fairly early times, of certain professional learned classes with a strong hereditary principle—bards, lawyers, and in Ireland and Scotland, families of doctors, like the O'Davorens, Hickeys and Livingstones. The evidence of the Welsh law books and the story of Meddygon Myddfai suggests that the same may be true, to a lesser extent, of Wales. The story of the Scottish Gaelic family of Beaton is well attested.[12] During the XIIIth century, a certain Mac Betha, anglicised Beaton or Macbeth, went to Scotland from Ireland as physician to Angus óg, Lord of the Isles. Descendants of Mac Betha continued to hold lands and practise medicine in Gaelic Scotland up until the XVIIIth century. One of the chief claims of this family to distinction was that they possessed Gaelic MSS containing Gaelic translations of classical medical texts—their reputation was largely based on the esoteric knowledge they gained from these books—which were assiduously copied and preserved in the family library. Edward Lhuyd, the greatest of Welsh scientists and antiquarians, saw some of their MSS when he visited one John Beaton in the early XVIIIth century.[13]

The Beaton story resembles strongly what we know of Meddygon Myddfai and spans much the same period. The Myddfai family claimed descent from Rhiwallon, whose patron was Rhys Gryg, Lord of Dinefwr ; the Beatons from Mac Betha, whose patron was Angus Ôg. Much store was placed on the value of their books. Edward Lhuyd, just as he looked with interest at the MSS of John Beaton, was an assiduous copier of Meddygon Myddfai texts.[14] What then were these books or texts ? The two colophons mentioned earlier suggest a twofold MS tradition. The one seems to be the prefix to a specific text for which Rhiwallon and his sons were responsible ; the second refers to collections derived from various books and possible accretions from various sources attributed to the canonical authority of Meddygon Myddfai. The MS history of vernacular medical texts in Welsh deriving from a medieval source is complicated. We should like to devote the rest of this paper to a short discussion of the three earliest MSS of which we know containing one or other or both of the colophons.

The earliest one, the Welsh School MS, now kept at the British Museum belongs to the second half of the XIVth century. A particularly interesting book on many accounts, we are more than grateful to Mr Philip Wyn Davies for the reference which led us to this text. It contains both colophons. The second is the text contained in the *Llyfr Coch Hergest,* a great golden treasury of medieval Welsh literature written about 1400. [This text has already been published by both Ab Ithel(1) and Diverres(2)]. The third, of roughly the same date, is a small MS XXII, in the Jesus College, Oxford Collections of MSS. We have listed and analysed the contents of all three.

THE MANUSCRIPTS

MS I

The earliest surviving MS, BM Add. MS 14,912 belongs to the second half of the XIVth century. During the XVIIIth century it was in the possession of the Welsh antiquary and man of learning, Lewis Morris.

The entry in the British Museum Catalogue reads as follows :

> Meddygon Myddfai, or the practise of Physic of the Myddvai Doctors, a collection of Recipes for various diseases and injuries, prognostics, charms, virtues of herbs etc. in Welsh by the physicians of Myddfai co. Caermarthen ;—Aristotles instructions to Alexander, on physiognomy etc., in Welsh :—Latin and Welsh vocabulary of herbs etc. A Welsh calendar is prefixed. On Vellum, written in the XIV C.

The MS is annotated and indexed in the hand of Lewis Morris and has additional scientific material in a seventeenth century hand. From Lewis Morris it passed into the Welsh School Collection and from there in 1843 into the British Museum. It has never been published.

Here is a list of contents :

Calendar
Fevers and their treatment*
Abdominal disorders*
List of days for blood-letting and diet in twelve months of the year*
Remedies (4)
Gynaecology, remedies (2)
Remedies (4)
The seven enemies of the eye*
Three broken bones which will never knit*
Remedies (2)
COLOPHON I*
The first thing to be discussed is the head*
Parts of the head and mention of craniotomy*
Diseases from head to lungs with remedies (6)*
Dysuria ; procedure for lithotomy*
Remedies (7)

....

Translations of *De Corio Serpentis* of Johannes Paulus by one Phylip
Days of month
COLOPHON II
Importance of knowledge of twelve signs of the Zodiac
Remedies (3) including *Rhad Duw* (Gratia Dei) and apothecary's measures
Soporific sponge[0]
Letter of Aristotle to Alexander the Great on physiognomy[0],

De secretis secretorum
The four elements and the four humours
Uroscopy*
Brief instructions for blood-letting*
Remedies and recipes (34)
The eight parts of a man*
The three thick indispensibles*
The three thin indispensibles*
The three lingering wounds*
Remedies and recipes (6)
The greatest and smallest remedies*
Remedies and recipes (45)
Virtues of the leek*, mustard, pepper, sea holly, purslane, parsley, hart's tongue, cress, lettuce, mint, garlic and betony
(8 missing leaves)
Judicial astrology in Latin
Remedies (7)
Virtues of the scabious, with part in Latin verse (from Macer Floridus)
Prognostications
Precepts
Latin instructions on preparing pills, poultices and physic
Latin-Welsh vocabulary of plant names.

MS II

The second text, contained in Jesus MS XCIX, *Llyfr Coch Hergest*, was written about 1400. This text has already been published twice; first by Ab Ithel, and secondly in the admirable edition of Pol Diverres *Le Plus ancien texte des Meddygon Myddveu*. The inclusion of a medical text in this great literary compendium which was written in south Wales possibly reflects a fashion of the late Middle Ages which considered a certain amount of medical knowledge to be the pre-requisite of any well educated noblemen. In Ireland, the Earl of Kildare in 1500 paid the equivalent of £1000 for the MS of an Irish medical textbook.

COLOPHON I
The first thing to be discussed is the head*
Parts of the head and mention of craniotomy*

Diseases from head to lungs with remedies (5)*
Fevers and their treatment*
Haemorrhoids, their ligation and remedy (1)
Abdominal Disorders*
Dysuria ; procedure for lithotomy*
Gynaecology, remedies (2)
Virtues of plants (5)
Dietetics
Remedies (24)
Three difficulties of a doctor
Remedy (1)
Seven enemies of the eye*
Three broken bones which will never knit*
Remedies (6)
Charm against fever
Remedies or preventives (19)
List of days for blood-letting and diet in the twelve months of the year*
Unfortunate (Egyptian) days
Remedies (41)
Virtues of the leek*
Remedies (3) including some animal recipes
Virtues of mustard
Uroscopy*
Brief instructions for blood-letting*
Remedies (9)
The three thick indispensibles*
The three thin indispensibles*
The three lingering wounds*
Remedies (3)
The greatest remedies*
The smallest remedies*
Materia medica describing plants (13) in Latin, attributed to Constantine
Remedies (11)
Mention of medical sources and the four elements, followed by principles of hygiene similar to the Regimen Sanitatis.

MS III

The third MS belonging to a date later in the XVth century is a small medical MS Jesus MS XXII.

COLOPHON II
Calendar, including days for bloodletting and ' Egyptian ' days
Letters of Aristotle to Alexander on hygiene—*De Sanitatis tuenda*
Letters of Aristotle to Alexander on physiognomy—*De secretis secretorum*[0] ; virtues of plants and various meats and drinks
"Soporific sponge"[0]
Recipes and remedies (5)
The four humours
Continuation of letter of Aristotle to Alexander discussing virtues of various foods.
Virtues of wheat, barley, etc.
Remedies (55)
Virtues of the leek*, remedies (2)
Virtues of meats, part of which corresponds to supra..

Anyone who is familiar with popular medieval medical collections in Latin or vernacular languages other than Welsh will immediately recognise old friends among the lists of contents, for most of the material can be traced to Latin *exempla*. Medieval medical knowledge and literature throughout Europe was very largely based on classical learning, either the learning which had filtered through without interruption in Western Europe from classical times, or that which was reintroduced from the east after the recovery of Greek texts from Arabic sources and the Aristotelian revival of the XIth and XIIth centuries. Popular collections deriving ultimately from this *materia medica* were in general a very mixed bunch.[15] These Welsh texts give a fair idea of the range. They consisted of collections of recipes which seemed to be common throughout Europe and were ultimately based on classical collections (the paragraphs listed remedies) deriving from lists of remedies for various diseases or from herbals describing the qualities of special plants ; short treatises or tracts describing commonly practised operations like the removal of bladder stone or lithotomy ; the magico-medical science of uroscopy, horoscopes, calendars indicating lucky or unlucky days for blood-letting and other treatments, instructions as to diet, rules for hygiene, texts deriving from the pseudo-Aristotelian literature of the XIIth and XIIIth centuries, like the letter of Aristotle to Alexander[16] and certain magico-alchemical texts like the *De Corio Serpentis* or the *Twelve Virtues of Snakeskin.*[17] Some of these tracts were available in Western Europe from an early date.

The *List of days for Blood-letting and diet in the Twelve Months of the Year* in the British Museum MS and *Llyfr Coch Hergest*, for instance, corresponds to a Latin List in a IXth century Chartres MS.[18] Other tractates derive from XIIth and XIIIth century Latin sources, like the *Letters of Aristotle* and the *Snakeskin Tract.* Some of this material was, doubtless, part of the oral teaching of the schools, and would be part of the repertoire of any doctor who had been in contact with them.

It is outside the compass of this paper to deal in detail with these Latin origins. We have indicated some of them by using Latin titles in the lists. The chief concern of this paper is with the family of Myddfai and the nature of the rules which they caused to be written down.

All three MSS which we are discussing derive from a period some 150 years after the time of Rhys Gryg, and in the nature of medieval texts, particularly medieval technical MSS, it would be unusual if their contents had remained unchanged. The contents of all three are far from identical. The first and earliest MS already contains two colophons ; the second the first colophon only ; the third the second colophon. The MS to which we wish to pay particular attention is the *British Museum MS,* referring to the other two for comparison. Internal orthographical evidence and the external evidence of another MS suggest that the contents of this book derive from at least two immediate sources. One source contained the material up to the dotted line ; the other the rest of the text. To take the contents of the second part first, apart from the snakeskin text and the horoscope, the rest of the list follows a copy of the second colophon. This list includes a number of short philosophical or scientific tracts like the one discussing the 'four elements' and the 'four humours' and the *Letters of Aristotle to Alexander the Great.* Apart from one of these letters, this part of the *British Museum MS* has very little in common with the contents of the third MS listed which is also preceded by a form of the second colophon. The items which are common are marked by o. The divergence suggests that these collections may owe very little to the original works of Meddygon Myddfai, but were tracts drawn to the canon of the doctors because of their reputation.

The contents of the first half of the MS which contain a copy of the first colophon may be compared with contents of the *Llyfr Coch Hergest* text preceded by a copy of the same colophon. Asterisks indicate items common to both MSS. The contents of the first part of both MSS are almost identical, although the order is somewhat different. In the *Llyfr Coch*, the colophon occurs at the beginning. We think that the *Llyfr Coch* order is probably the correct one, and that the order in the *British Museum MS* has been confused. One of the fundamental orders of describing disease in classical medical texts was one which began with the top of the head. The colophon in both MSS is followed by a statement which suggests derivation of some such order. ' First of all we shall treat of the head, for that is the chief part of man's body '. In the *Llyfr Coch* the first five items, excluding the stray ' Haemorrhoid ' remedy, which does not occur in the Welsh School text, follow the head-downwards order.

A treatise of this nature might well have formed the nucleus of Rhiwallon's composition. Perhaps there were other tracts in it like the following ones in the *Llyfr Coch Hergest*. Further studies and comparisons of other MSS will, we hope, bring more light on the subject.[19]

On December 29th, 1760, Lewis Morris, that erudite Welsh scholar and man of science, was writing to his brother Richard with a copy of the British Museum MS before him.

> Oni ddywedasoch i mai Doctor phisig yw Doctor Owen ? A glywodd ef erioed sôn am Feddygon Myddfai ?
> An account of that MS of the Britains will be a good subject of a letter to the Cymmrodorion.[20]

The letter never seems to have been written, or if it was, has not been preserved. If it had been, this paper would doubtless have been unnecessary.

NOTES

1 Ab Ithel, J. W. (ed.) *The Physicians of Myddvai,* Roderic, for Welsh MSS Society, Llandovery, 1861.

2 Diverres, P., *Le Plus Ancien Texte des Meddygon Myddveu,* Le Dault, Paris, 1913, p. xxviii.

3 Ab Ithel, op. cit. ; Diverres, *op. cit.* ; also transcripts of Myddfai Parish Records in N.L.W. and gravestone in the Church at Myddfai.

4 Davies, H., *Welsh Botanology,* The Author, London, 1813, p. vii.

5 *Welsh Med. Gaz.,* Cardiff 1971 (Winter).

6 Lloyd, J. E., *History of Wales,* 3rd ed. Longman, London 1939, Vol. II, p. 768.

7 Rees, William, *An Historical Atlas of Wales,* 2nd ed., Faber, London, 1959.

8 Smith, J. Beverley, 'The "Chronica De Wallia" and the Dynasty of Dinefwr,' *Bull. Bd. celtic stud.* (1963), 20, 261-282.

9 Cule, John, The Court Mediciner and Medicine in the Laws of Wales, *J. Hist Med.* (1966) 21, 213-236.

10 Richard, A. J., 'Castles, Boroughs and Religious Houses', Chapter 4 in J. E. Lloyd, *History of Carmarthenshire,* Lewis, Cardiff, 1935, Vol. I, p. 322.

11 Edwards, J. Goronwy, *The Normans and the Welsh March,* Raleigh Lecture in History, *Proc. Br. Acad.* (1956), 42, 155-177.

12 Thomson, Derick S., 'Gaelic Learned Orders and Literati in Mediaeval Scotland. *Proceedings of the Third International Congress of Celtic Studies.* (*Scott. Stud.,* 12, 57-78), ed. W. F. H. Nicolaisen School of Scottish Studies, Edinburgh, 1968 ; D. Mackinnon, 'The Genealogy of the Macbeths or Beatons of Islay and Mull', *Caledon. med. J.,* (1902), 5, 141-153.

13 Campbell, J. L., and Thomson, D. S., (eds.), *Edward Lhuyd in the Scottish Highlands* 1699-1700, Clarendon Press, Oxford, 1963, p. 9ff.

14 The Medical MSS Peniarth 119 and Peniarth 120E were copied by or for Edward Lhuyd and he owned Bodleian Rawlinson B467.

15 Sigerist, H. E., 'Materia medica in the Middle Ages', *Bull. Hist. of Med.,* (1939), 7, 417-423.

16 Thorndike, Lynn P., *A History of Magic and Experimental Science,* Vol. 2, Macmillan, New York, 1923, p. 246ff.

17 Williams, Ifor, 'Rhinweddau Croen Neidr', *Bull. Bd. Celtic Stud.* (1927) 4, J. W. S. Johnsson, 'Les Experimenta duodecim Johannis Paulini (De Corio Serpentis)', *Bull. Soc. fr. Hist. Méd.,* (1913), 12, 257-267.

18 Wickersheimer, Ernest, 'Textes Médicaux Chartrains des IXe, Xe et XIe siècles', *Science, Medicine and History,* ed. by E. A. Underwood, Oxford University Press, London 1953, Vol. I, p. 171.

19 Mr Gerallt Harries has described other hereditary physicians, the family of Bened Feddyg in Denbighshire, elsewhere in these Proceedings. A fuller account of the Meddygon Myddfai tradition and manuscripts is due to appear in *Studia Celtica.*

20 J. H. Davies, (ed.), *The Letters of Lewis, Richard, William and John Morris of Anglesey,* 1728-1765, The Editor, Aberystwyth, 1909, vol. II, p. 284.

BENED FEDDYG: A WELSH MEDICAL PRACTITIONER IN THE LATE MEDIEVAL PERIOD

W. GERALLT HARRIES

The Welsh medieval medical manuscripts which have survived the ravages of time are conspicuous by their paucity.[1] The earliest of those which are extant belong to the late fourteenth and early fifteenth centuries.[2] As in the case of so many of its other records, both literary and non-literary, Wales has lost much of its written medical lore, through neglect and sheer misfortune.[3]

Another regrettable fact is that we know very little about the practitioners who compiled, or who commissioned the compiling of, our medieval medical manuscripts. Four of these manuscripts[4] claim that their contents are partly based on the teachings of the famous practitioners of Myddfai, in north-east Carmarthenshire, but it is impossible to discover the names of the compilers or original owners of these codices.[5] A few of our late medieval compilations are known to be the work of clerical practitioners,[6] but it is far more difficult to identify the lay practitioners who must have produced similar works. The names of many lay practitioners of medicine in medieval Wales have been preserved for us in the extant records of the period,[7] but these names cannot be associated with any known medical writings.

In the light of these several considerations, the discovery of a medical manuscript which was compiled or owned by a lay practitioner in Wales, even in the late medieval period, is a rare and rather notable event. One such manuscript is Sotheby MS C.2., which is now preserved in the National Library of Wales, Aberystwyth. Its original owner, whose name appears in the manuscript as Bened ap Rhys[8] and Bened Feddyg,[9] was a practitioner in the Vale of Clwyd, Denbighshire. Various holograph entries throughout the manuscript reveal that the compilation was transmitted from father to son, and that it remained in the possession of Bened's family for at least three generations after his death. During this period it was considerably enlarged by a number of unidentified practitioners or scribes, who augmented the original work with additional treatises and recipes.

The holograph additions and notes by Bened's direct descendants deserve a little attention. His son William wrote his name on two separate pages[10] in a small, neat, round hand, and he inserted recipes and other medical material in several places.[11] The hand of William's son, Hugh, is identified by his signature on two pages of the manuscript;[12] this identification establishes the authorship of an interesting note,[13] in the same hand, which informs us that the manuscript was (or, perhaps, would be at a future date) 'the book of Huw ap William ap Bened after his father', and adds, 'Hughe ap William was a year old... [in the year] 1528.' The last member of the family whose name is recorded in the manuscript is Hugh's son, John; he entered his signature on three separate pages,[14] and stated that the book was in his possession. John's statement is corroborated and amplified by two notes in the manuscript, in a distinctive hand which is clearly that of Thomas Evans of Hendreforfudd, a well-known contemporary poet and scribe with a taste for medical lore. One note[15] confirms that on January the 16th, 1616 (=1617), the manuscript was 'the book of John ap Huw ap Wiliam ap Bened ap Rhys of Llanelidan,' while the other[16] records that John was born 'in the second year after Queen Mary's coronation' and that he had, therefore attained the age of sixty-seven in 1621.

On the basis of these facts, gleaned from the family manuscript, and of evidence which has been preserved in a few Welsh genealogical manuscripts of the sixteenth and early seventeenth centuries, it is possible to identify Bened Feddyg. His pedigree was briefly recorded[17] by the renowned Welsh bard and genealogist, Simwnt Fychan (d. 1606), who lived in the neighbouring parish of Llanfair Dyffryn Clwyd. Simwnt was a contemporary of Bened's grandson, Huw ab Wiliam, and we can safely assume that they knew each other well, as they shared a common interest in Welsh poetry and music. The genealogical evidence testifies to Bened's noble lineage; he could claim descent (through Heilin Frych) from Marchweithian, the founder of one of the fifteen noble tribes of Gwynedd. His wife, Annes, was of a social status equal to that of her husband; she could trace her pedigree to Rhirid Du, and thence to Llywelyn Eurdorchog of Yale, the founding father of a considerable number of proud families in north-east Wales. It is almost certain that she was a native of Llanelidan or a neighbouring parish ; most of the descendants of Rhirid Du seem to have settled in that area. Bened's family origins, on the other hand, must be sought in the hundred of Isaled, in the northern half of Denbighshire ; his relatives dwelt mainly in the parishes of Henllan and Llannefydd. One is tempted to suggest that he was a native of Isaled and that he settled in Llanelidan after his marriage ; in the absence of supporting evidence, however, this must remain an unsubstantiated theory.

Of Bened's son, William, we know nothing other than his name. It seems that he inherited his father's interest in medicine, and he also may have been a practitioner, at least on a part-time basis.[18] In the case of William's son, Hugh, we can offer a brief biography. He was born, as we have seen, in 1527, and we have documentary evidence that he was still alive in 1581.[19] His accomplishments as a harpist were praised by five contemporary Welsh poets.[20] Hugh was also deeply interested in bardic poetry, and a four-line stanza, known as an *englyn*, composed by him, reveals that he had mastered the basic elements of the Welsh strict-metre system.[21] A well-known manuscript collection of Welsh poetry[22] contains two specific references to him, and that manuscript may well have been in his possession at one time.

In the light of the evidence which is available, particularly the dates of birth of his grandson and great-grandson, it would seem safe to assume that Bened was born about 1470–1480. A number of important questions concerning his career seem to be unanswerable. We can do no more than ponder unprofitably on the nature and extent of his medical training and education : we should like to know whether he received a formal education[23] or whether he was merely apprenticed to another local practitioner. The only evidence, in the apparent absence of other relevant records, on which we can form an opinion of Bened as a practitioner is the manuscript which he once possessed. It is very likely that he treated it as a text-book ; he may, of course, have had access to other compilations which have not been preserved. There can be no doubt that he held in high esteem the treatises and recipes which found a place in his compilation, and it seems reasonable to suggest that they formed the basis on which he diagnosed the ailments of those who resorted to him and prescribed remedies for them.

The manuscript, in its present form, is a composite one, and it is imperfect in several places. Three broad sections are readily identifiable. The first of these, which occupies the first 132 of the manuscript's 242 pages, is entirely in one hand, and there can be no doubt that this comprises Bened's original compilation. It has been foliated throughout by the original scribe,[24] who also appended a complete list of the contents.[25] The gaps in the foliation reveal the fact that nine folios have been lost, while the index provides us with a guide to the contents of those missing folios. It is quite apparent that this first section of the present manuscript is an entity, and it must have the first claim on our attention when we attempt to offer an assessment of Bened as a practitioner.

Bened's book is a carefully planned and well-ordered compilation,[26] derived from various medieval sources. The first text is a treatise on the four humours which constitute a man's body and govern his 'complexion'.[27] It serves as an introduction to a much longer treatise on the nature and properties of various foods and beverages, in so far as they relate to the four humours.[28] These treatises were probably the handbook which Bened consulted before formulating his dietary prescriptions. The first lacuna in the text has denied us the end of the treatise on foods and beverages, as well as the greater part of a discourse on pulse taking.[29] The next treatise discusses the sun, the moon, the twelve winds and the planets, and defines their place in the humoral hypothesis.[30] The remainder of the compilation consists almost entirely of a substantial collection of recipes,[31] amounting to almost three hundred separate items. The compiler, who attributed the remedies to the two great authorities of the ancient world, 'Volusianus' and Aristotle,[32] included a systematic selection of remedies for ailments in various parts of the body and described the method of preparing a number of ointments, electuaries, poultices and plasters, some of which were specific, while others were panaceas. Two short treatises find a place amongst the recipes; one is an abbreviated version of a well-known tract on uroscopy,[33] and the other is a brief statement of the general principles of phlebotomy,[34] which is attributed to 'Volusian,' who is described as the greatest master of the art after Aristotle. We are later reminded that the work is based on the teachings of 'Volusianus' and Aristotle,[35] and 'Macer's book'[36] is recommended as a guide to the properties of herbs. The only other authorities referred to are Hippocrates, the reputed source of a remedy for the palsy,[37] and Ptolemy, whose opinion is quoted on the importance of considering the planetary conjunctions of the moon when administering certain remedies.[38] The remaining items are words of general advice to a medical apprentice,[39] a short treatise, attributed to Aristotle, on the four parts of the human body, which are related to the four elements,[40] a treatise on palmistry,[41] a long Christian charm,[42] and, finally, a copy of the Latin version of the Proem to St John's Gospel, written in Welsh orthography.[43] The list of contents completes this first section of our manuscript.

The second section consists of a long treatise, in English, on uroscopy,[44] preceded by a partial translation into Welsh.[45] The writer was one Tudur ab Elise, and his colophon[46] establishes the fact that he wrote during Bened's lifetime. He may have been apprenticed to Bened or merely employed by him as a scribe. We can safely assume that this treatise, on a subject of primary importance to a medieval practitioner, was available to Bened, and that he consulted it for the purposes of diagnosis and prognosis.

It is difficult to draw a precise line of demarcation between the second and third sections of the manuscript. The twenty-two pages following the English treatise on uroscopy should probably be considered as part of the second section, as they contain a number of items which were written in the early part of the sixteenth century. These include tables,[47] a treatise on uroscopy in Welsh,[48] a rough sketch of the human hand indicating the chief lines,[49] and two further contributions by Tudur ab Elise.[50] Examples of later hands, mainly of the sixteenth century, are found on many of these pages.

The third, and final section of Sotheby MS C.2. is a miscellaneous assortment of material, mainly medical or quasi-medical, in a variety of hands which were roughly contemporary with Bened's son and grandson. The contents of these pages reflect William ap Bened's amateur, if not professional, commitment to medicine, and they bear witness also to his son Hugh's taste for bardic poetry. The first text is a well-organised treatise,[51] in the hand of a good penman, on the seven planets, the four elements and the four 'complexions'. It also discusses the relationship between the four humours and the four seasons of the year, and lists the so-called 'dogs' days' which, it was believed, were governed by the planet Canicula Canis, and the 'Egyptian days', of which all medieval physicians took careful note before prescribing phlebotomy. The treatise ends with a short regimen for the four seasons. The same scribe appends a cognate text,[52] which I have identified as a translation into Welsh of the first prologue to the well-known book, *Le Compost et Kalendrier des Bergiers*, which was first published in Paris in 1493 and reprinted several times during the sixteenth century. The book was equally popular in the English versions, the first of which appeared in 1503. Two other texts in the latter part of the manuscript deserve mention, each in the hand of a different scribe. The first is a regimen for the different months of the year,[53] which, like other medieval guides to good health, was probably derived, through the Salernitan regimen, from the treatment of the subject in the *Corpus Hippocraticum*. The other text is a partial translation into Welsh of the immensely popular *Secretum Secretorum*,[54] which was wrongly ascribed to Aristotle in the Middle Ages. Modern scholars inform us that the work, which was compiled from different sources, had assumed something like its present form by about the seventh or eighth centuries A.D. It was translated into Latin, from Arabic, on two occasions between the twelfth and thirteenth centuries, —firstly by John of Spain (Johannes Hispalensis), and, secondly, by one Philip, a cleric.[55] We know that a partial translation into Welsh had appeared by the second half of the fourteenth century, as it is included in our oldest medical manuscript,[56] which was compiled during that period. A number of poems, in the Welsh strict metres, have been written on blank pages, or portions of pages, towards the end of the manuscript.[57] They are in the hand of an unidentified scribe, probably a contemporary of Bened's grandson, Huw ab Wiliam, whose inclinations and interests, as we have already observed, probably account for their inclusion in the manuscript.

It is apparent, from this brief survey of the contents of Sotheby MS C.2., that Bened was a compiler in the true medieval tradition, as, indeed, were the unidentified persons who added their contributions to form the present manuscript. A considerable number of manuscripts, containing similar material to that found in Bened's book, has survived in Britain and on the Continent ; many were written in Latin, and some, especially from the fourteenth century onwards, in the vernacular languages. This basic similarity between medieval medical manuscripts, in spite of all the variations which we find on close examination, derives from the fact that they are all ultimately based on the medical theory which Galen propounded in his numerous works. Galen accepted the humoral theory, which he found in the Hippocratic writings, as well as the 'doctrine of contraries' or the theory of treatment by opposites. The underlying principle of his diagnostic method was that diseases were caused by a deficiency of one or more of the four humours. He maintained[58] that all substances possess the same hot, cold, dry and moist qualities as are present in a healthy human body, and that these qualities are found in four degrees of intensity. The system was varied, to a greater or lesser extent, by many writers and compilers during the Dark and Middle Ages, but one can safely assert that its essential features were preserved and that it was the greatest single influence on medical theory throughout the medieval period. Systematic lists of the qualities and degrees of materia medica are found in several of the well-known works of the period, such as the *Inventarium seu collectorium cyrurgie* of Guy de Chauliac.[59] This of course, is the basis of the classification of foods according to their humoral content in the treatise which is found in Bened's manuscript, as well as in earlier Welsh compilations.

The Galenic diagnostic theory pervades the recipe literature of the Middle Ages. It is usually tacitly assumed rather than categorically stated. In many cases the compilers were not even aware of the fact that the recipes conformed with the theory, as they had inherited most of them from earlier compilers. There was, in fact, a long recipe tradition, which can certainly be traced as far back as ancient Egypt,[60] and it contained much pre-Galenic material, such as recipes found in in the works of Hippocrates, Celsus, Dioscorides, the elder Pliny[61] and others. Many of these earlier recipes were later embodied in Galen's own works, but he modified them to conform to his own teaching. The recipes were further modified and augmented by later compilers. In the five centuries subsequent to Galen's death (*c.* 200 A.D.) we find a number of writers whose compilations had a considerable influence on the recipe tradition ; some of the most well-known of these were Apuleius Barbarus, Sextus Placitus, Alexander of Tralles, and Paul of Aegina. Later compilations, such as the Anglo-Saxon Leechbooks, reveal the Christianizing of pagan charms and magical cures.[62] An important new source of recipes was absorbed into the European tradition when the medical works of the Arabs were translated into Latin in the eleventh and twelfth centuries. The Arabic physicians, such as Rhazes, Haly Abbas and Avicenna, had drawn not only on the Hippocratic and Galenic tradition, but also on Eastern sources for their materia medica, and they were expert pharmacists.

Their syrups, salves and electuaries were now introduced into Europe, especially by a group of physicians who practised at Salernum,[63] of whom Constantinus Africanus was one of the most famous.

These, then, were the ultimate sources of medieval European medicine, and, thus, of Bened's book. The immediate channels through which some of the elements of this long tradition reached his compilation are difficult, if not, indeed, impossible to determine. An abundance of parallels can be located, particularly in the five earliest extant Welsh medical compilations.[64] These parallels are often so close, amounting in some cases to an almost exact correspondence, even in the wording, that we are led to the conclusion that Bened's immediate sources were mainly, if not entirely, written in the Welsh language. A comparative study of our earliest extant texts reveals a host of examples of close agreement, as well as many points of divergence, and on this evidence we are obliged to suggest that a corpus of written medical material had been amassed in Wales by the middle of the fourteenth century, at the latest. This corpus, which seems never to have been codified, was constantly augmented as new treatises and recipes became available in the Welsh language. It was the main source of our medical compilations, which reflect not only the volume of material which comprised the corpus at the point in time when the compilation was made but also the proportion of it which was available to the compiler.

We have already referred to the fact that the treatises on the four humours and on the properties of foods in Bened's book are found, with variations, in earlier Welsh manuscripts, and that his treatise on uroscopy seems to be an abbreviated version of one that occurs in earlier compilations,[65] Other examples of close agreement, which indicate that Bened's immediate sources included much of the material which is found in our earliest medical collections, include a treatment for strangury, incorporating a procedure for lithotomy,[66] a discourse on craniotomy,[67] a method of prognosticating whether or not a patient's illness is fatal,[68] and three medical triads.[69] There is also a plenitude of parallels to many of the recipes offered by Bened. Exact parallels can be cited to his remedies for an aposteme,[70] for 'proud flesh',[71] for bad breath,[72] for the bladder stone,[73] for haemorrhoids,[74] for goitre,[75] for abdominal hardness or swelling,[76] for lung sores,[77] and for ringworm caused by a 'wet humour',[78] as well as to the method which he records of preventing drunkenness[79] and of staunching blood.[80] Many of his salves or ointments, some of which are described as panaceas, were known in Wales before his time.[81] His book includes a copy of the prologue to a well-known medieval recipe for an entrete, or plaster, to which the Welsh versions gave the name *Rhad Duw* (God's Grace[82]) It was usually known in the compilations of other countries by its Latin name, *Gratia Dei,*[83] although the variant *Donum Dei* does occur.[84] One, at least, of Bened's recipes is recorded in an earlier Welsh manuscript as a prescription for a different condition.[85]

The parallels, as we should expect, are not confined to earlier Welsh collections. For a sty, or a web in the eye, Bened offers a remedy which contains elements frequently found in a wide variety of earlier remedies for eye disorders. His recipe,[86] which consists of the gall of a goat, the gall of a hare, the gall of a red cockerel, and the celandine, is made up of ingredients which may be found in a host of earlier eye remedies. The celandine is one of the plants listed in the Salernitan regimen as being beneficial to the eyes,[87] while animal gall had been used from the Biblical and Classical periods for treating various eye conditions.[88] Another of Bened's eye remedies prescribes the centaury.[89] It is interesting to note that the Welsh name for this plant is *bustl y ddaear* (' the earth's gall '). Bened records this fact, and there can be little doubt that he, and other Welsh physicians, regarded it as the counterpart, in the plant world, of the efficacious animal gall. One other parallel must suffice for our present purpose, The tokens of death listed by Bened[90] contain many of the items found in a similar list in a fifteenth century English manuscript.[91] Some of these can be traced back to the Salernitan Collection, and thence to Avicenna, Celsus, and even Hippocrates in his *Prognosticon*.

Bened Feddyg was probably not aware of these and many other parallels which could be cited, and it is very likely that he would have been surprised to hear of them. He seems to have accepted without question that the treatises and recipes which he had gathered from older sources[92] constituted the distilled wisdom of the ancients ; this he regarded as a priceless heritage, which should, at all costs, be preserved amongst the initiated. It was not for him to question this authoritative body of learning ; in the entire compilation we find no hint of experimentation or of doubt (based upon his experience as a practitioner) about the efficacy of any traditional remedies. In this, as well as in other respects, Bened was, in all probability, a fairly typical representative of the medical practitioners of rural Wales in the early sixteenth century. On the evidence afforded by his manuscript, he seems hardly distinguishable, in his practice of medicine, from his predecessors in the fourteenth and fifteenth centuries. The earlier treatises and remedies were still adequate for him, and he reveals no apparent desire for change or modification. The picture, admittedly, is sketchy and imperfect, but it does seem to reveal that Bened and his colleagues in similar circumstances constituted a stagnant and backward-looking profession.

NOTES

The following abbreviations are used for the texts which are most frequently cited :

B.M.—B.M.Add. MS 14912.

H—Havod MS 16 (in the Cardiff Central Library ; this text has been edited by Miss Ida B. Jones, *Revue Celtique:* Vol. VII (1955-6), pp. 46-75, 270-339, and Vol. VIII (1958-9), pp. 66-97, 346-393.

Hens.—G. Henslow : *Medical Works of the Fourteenth Century* (London 1899).

J.—Jesus College MS 22 (in the Bodleian Library, Oxford).

M.M.—P. Diverres : *Le plus ancien texte de Meddygon Myddfeu* (Paris, 1913). (This work publishes the text of Jesus College MS 111, known as the Red Book of Hergest, cols. 928-959).

Rawl.—Rawlinson MS B. 467 (in the Bodleian Library, Oxford).

Soth.—Sotheby MS C.2. (in the National Library of Wales, Aberystwyth).

Th.—M.S. Ogden (ed.) : *The 'Liber de Diversis Medicinis' in the Thornton Manuscript* (E.E.T.S., Orig. Series, no. 207), 1938.

1 This does not seem to have been the case at the beginning of the eighteenth century. Edward Lhuyd, in the catalogue of Welsh manuscripts which he published in his *Archaeologia Britannica* (Oxford, 1707), states (p. 262, *sub* 'Medhygon Mydhvei') : *Alii etiam in hoc Genere extant Codices MSS non pauci.*

2 A palaeographical examination of B.M. leads one to suggest that it was probably written in the third quarter of the fourteenth century. The date which has been assigned to both H. and the Red Book text (=M.M.) is *circa* 1400 (Hist. MSS Comm., *Report on MSS in the Welsh Lang.*, Vol. II, pt. 2, 1902, pp. 1, 318), while J. has been placed in the 'late XVth century' (*ibid.*, p. 38),—a dating which may be rather late. Unlike the others, Rawl. is a composite MS. Fols 1 *recto*-15 *verso* were probably written about, or soon after, 1400 ; the other hands in this MS are a little later in the fifteenth century. In one respect, Rawl. is the most interesting of these five MSS. A note on the inner side of the front cover, in the hand of Edward Lhuyd, states : '*Edvardo Luidio donavit D. T. Thomas á Cwr y*

Wayn apud Maridunenses. Anno 1698'. Lhuyd refers to the MS and the donor in the same location as the extract cited above (n.1), and adds that Cwr-y waun is near the town of Llangadog, in the Vale of Towy. In fact, Cwr-y-waun (locally known as Cwr-weun) is near the road which leads from Llangadog to Myddfai, and is within easy reach of the reputed homes of the renowned Meddygon Myddfai. One is, therefore, tempted to suggest that the MS, or, at least, a part of it, was written in the vicinity of Myddfai.

3 Two notable examples of this misfortune come readily to mind. Fires at Hafod Uchtryd, Cardiganshire (13th March, 1807) and Wynnstay, near Ruabon, Denbighshire (5th to 6th March, 1858), destroyed a large number of the manuscripts in these two fine private libraries, each of which held a good proportion of the manuscripts collected by Edward Lhuyd (n. 1 *supra*). We know from early catalogues of these libraries that each of them contained a number of medical manuscripts.

4 B.M., fols. 20 *recto* & 31 *verso* ; M.M., p.6 ; Rawl., fol. 17 *verso* ; J., pp. 1-2.

5 It is interesting to note that later readers or owners of B.M. include the fifteenth century bard, Dafydd Nanmor (his name occurs twice, viz., at the tops of fols. 16 *recto* and 61 *recto*, in a hand which is identical with his signature in the Book of Aneirin) ; the sixteenth century humanist and reformer, William Salesbury (I feel confident that *marginalia* on fols. 20 *recto*, 52 *verso*—54 *recto*, 57 *recto*, 61 *verso*, and 72 *verso* are in his distinctive hand) ; and the eighteenth century poet and scholar, Lewis Morris, who provided the manuscript with a title-page and a list of contents as well as a number of notes. H. contains a number of *marginalia* in the hand of Dafydd Benwyn, a sixteenth century Glamorgan bard (on pp. 7, 23, 24, 27, 67, 69, 81, 82, 84, 88, 95, 97 and 98) ; other entries suggest that this manuscript remained in Glamorgan throughout the sixteenth and seventeenth centuries.

6 Examples are *Sir* Hugh Pennant, who wrote Peniarth MS 182, about 1514, and Dafydd ap Griffith, *effyriad* (a cleric), who wrote Llanstephan MS 10 in 1515.

7 E.g., Einion Goch, *ffisegor:* and Madog Veddyg, who were residents of Newborough, Anglesey, in 1352 (*The Record of Caernarvon,* ed. Sir Henry Ellis, 1838, p. 85) ; Eynon *physicus,* of Bangor (*ibid,* p. 92) ; and Grono Vethyk, of the townships of Dwygraig and Maestran in the commote of Penllyn in Merioneth, in 1419-20 (*ibid.*, p 262). The names of Ynyr ap Madog Feddyg and Simon ap Madog Feddyg are recorded in the Caernarvon Court Rolls for the 17th. May, 1371, and the 3rd March, 1402, respectively (G. P. Jones and Hugh Owen, eds., *Caernarvon Court Rolls,* 1361-1402, Caerns. Hist. Soc. Records Series, No. I, 1951, pp. 62, 176). A practitioner named Dafydd Feddyg is located in Flintshire in the late fourteenth century ; his son, Madog ap Dafydd Feddyg is listed as a freeholder in the township of Llys-y-coed (in the present parish of Cilcain) in the Ministers' Accounts for Flintshire in 1407 (Peniarth MS 287, p.xxx). Another practitioner, one Ieuan Feddyg, resided in the town or in the vicinity of Pwllheli, Caernarvonshire, in the middle of the fifteenth century ; one of his grandsons, Moris ap Gruffudd ab Ieuan Feddyg, was a

witness to deed drawn up at Pwllheli on Oct. 28, 1502 (N.L.W. Dolfrïog Deeds and Documents, no. 119), and another grandson, Morgan ap Gruffudd ab Ieuan Feddyg, acted in a similar capacity in the same town on August 4, 1509 (*ibid.*, no. 195).

8 In a Christian charm, on p. 116, we find the following supplication: *Christus ab omni malo defendat me Bened ap Res.* The fact that Bened's name is cited in the charm, in place of the customary impersonal *N* (=nomen), as, e.g., in H., p.19, and Th., 18, 57, suggests very forcibly that he actually wrote this copy of the charm. If this was the case, the first section of the manuscript (pp. 4-132) is entirely in his hand.

9 A colophon on p. 150, at the end of a treatise on uroscopy, reads thus: *Explicit liber Bened Veddig. Ed*idit *Tudur Ap Elisse.*

10 Once on p. 3 and four times on p. 211. He varies the form of his name from William/Wyllyam ap Benett to Wyllyam/William Benett.)

11 P. 3, containing five recipes, is entirely in his hand. He entered two recipes on p. 100, another two on p. 110, and five on p. 225. On p. 237 he listed a number of Welsh plant names and recorded the so-called 'perilous days'.

12 Pp. 1 and 227.

13 P. 110. The Welsh counterparts of the words 'the book of Huw ap' have been covered by a heavy stain—possibly in an attempt to delete them.

14 Pp. 39, 157 and 183. Also, a test for virginity, added at the foot of p. 189, may be in his hand.

15 P. 186.

16 P. 174.

17 Cardiff MS 4.265, fol. 301 *recto.*

18 Bened himself may have been a part-time practitioner. It seems reasonable to suggest that the practice of medicine in medieval Wales, particularly in the rural areas, was pursued on a part-time basis, in conjunction with another occupation, especially farming.

19 Amongst the deeds and documents which form the Welsh portion of the Crosse of Shaw Hill Collection, deposited at the National Library of Wales, there is an estreat from the court roll of the commote of Llannerch, in the lordship of Dyffryn Clwyd, recording the surrender of lands in four townships (situated in the parishes of Llanfair Dyffryn Clwyd and Llanelidan) by two parties (one of whom is named as Hugh ap William Benet) to the use of a third party. The estreat was taken on April 7th., 1581 (Crosse of Shaw Hill deed no. 980). Another deed (no. 250) in the same collection may refer to a daughter. It records the grant, in fee-farm, of a messuage in the township of Nantclwyd (in the parish of Llanelidan) to 'Elizabeth verch Hugh ap William of Nantcloyd, widow', on April 8th, 1612.

20 Peniarth MS 313, p. 40; Mostyn MS. 131, pp. 323-4, 352. The poets were Robert Evans, Thomas Evans, Siôn Mawddwy, Wiliam ap Robert and Siôn Meirion.

21 Peniarth MS. 313, p. 183.

22 Cardiff MS (=11), which is in two volumes. On p. 54 of the second volume Hugh's pedigree is briefly recorded, beneath an *englyn* which may,

perhaps, have been composed by him. On p. 30 of the same volume we find another *englyn*, which, we are told, was the work of ' a girl in her sleep '. The writer adds this statement about the source of his information : ' as hughe ap William sayth ali[a]s bened '.

23 His garbled versions of the names of two classical authors (notes 32 and 61) would seem to suggest that he received little, if any, formal education, particularly in medicine.

24 Fols. 1–67. It is very likely that Bened was the scribe (see note 8).

25 Pp. 117–132. These pages have not been foliated.

26 It is fairly clear that our earliest surviving medical manuscripts were compilations, rather than ' straight transcripts ' of other manuscripts in their entirety. Compilers either selected material from the sources which were available to them or, in some cases, included all or most of the medical and quasi-medical lore to which they had access. It would, therefore, be a misleading and profitless exercise to attempt to establish an arbitrary ' standard text ' of, for instance, those manuscripts which claim to record some of the teachings of the practitioners of Myddfai. In the absence of any surviving exemplar, which, in its entirety, could have served as his immediate source, we shall assume that Bened's book is a compilation, in the medieval tradition.

27 Pp. 4–7. Parallels are found in H., pp. 71–3, Rawl., fols. 1 *recto*–2 *verso* (impft.) and J., pp. 103–114.

28 Pp. 7–31. It is to be found also in H., pp. 11–14, 63–6, 73–80 (impft.) ; Rawl., fols. 2 *verso*–15 *verso* (impft.) ; J., pp. 66–93, 114–9, 157–162.

29 Five folios have been lost between p. 22 and p. 31.

30 Pp. 32–9.

31 Pp. 41–110.

32 This name, which occurs also on p. 101 (where he is described as ' chief physician to Caesar ') and p. 108 in the forms Volusian and Volusianus, presents us with a problem of identification. It is evidently a scribal error, possibly perpetuating an earlier scribal error. There seems to be no record of a physician bearing this name in classical times ; two persons named Volusianus found a place in the chronicles of the third century A.D.— one became Caesar and Augustus, while the other was a Praetorian Prefect (S. A. Cook *et al.: The Cambridge Ancient History*, Vol. XII, 1939, pp. 167, 183). It is a temptation to suggest, on the basis of the form Volusian, that the compiler is referring to the renowned Arab physician, Avicenna, whose name frequently appears in Europe in the form Avicien in the medieval period. However, the name normally associated with Aristotle and Hippocrates in medieval medical manuscripts is that of Galen, (cf. H., p. 29), to whom English compilers frequently refer eulogistically as ' the prince of leeches ' and ' the lantern of physicians and surgeons '. It is likely, therefore, that his name, which occurs in medieval manuscripts in such forms as Galenus, Galienus, Galen and Galien, was confused by Bened or one of his predecessors.

33 Pp. 67–9. A fuller version is found in B.M., fols. 54 *recto*–58 *recto* ; M.M., pp. 104–118 ; and H., pp. 91–4.

34 Pp. 101–2.
35 P. 108.
36 This was the hexameter poem, on the pharmaceutical powers of certain herbs, attributed throughout the Middle Ages, when it enjoyed immense popularity, to a tenth century herbalist, Macer Floridus, but now believed to be the work of Odo Magdunensis, a French physician. A printed version, under the title, *De herbarum virtutibus,* was published at Basle in 1527. One of the poem's hexameters (describing the reputed virtues of the Scabious) finds a place in B.M., fol. 81 *recto,* and the Latin text is glossed with a Welsh translation.
37 P. 51. An identical version is found in B.M., fols. 45 *recto* and *verso.*
38 P. 90.
39 P. 108.
40 Pp. 108–110.
41 Pp. 111–4. This is a version of a popular medieval treatise, of which the earliest copy of a Welsh version occurs in Peniarth MS 51, pp. 39–45 (in the hand of Gwilym Tew, *circa* 1450). A Middle English version of a broadly similar treatise on this subject was edited by Dr Hardin Craig in *The Works of John Metham* (E.E.T.S. Orig. Series, no. 132, 1906), pp. 84–117.
42 Pp. 115–6. Cf. n.8.
43 Pp. 116–7. The Proem to St John's Gospel (Chap. I, vv. 1–14), widely known by its opening words, *In principio,* was the object of special devotion from the days of the Christian Fathers, and was appointed as the gospel for Easter Day by the Eastern Church and by the Western Church as the gospel for Christmas Day. It was much abused during the Middle Ages. Mendicant friars and limitours used to recite it when begging—e.g., Chaucer's Friar (F. N. Robinson, ed., *The Complete Works of Geoffrey Chaucer,* Oxford, 1957, p. 19, ll. 253–5). It was also looked upon as a charm to exorcise devils, to drive away bad dreams, and to cure epilepsy (which was often known as *morbus Sancti Johannis*). This practice was certainly common by the twelfth century. Giraldus Cambrensis (*Opera*, ed. J. S. Brewer, Rolls Series, 1862, Vol. II, p. 129) states that the ignorant folk of his day believed in the exorcising powers of the *In principio.* For a fuller treatment of the subject see R. A. Law in *P.M.L.A.,* Vol. XXXVII (1922), pp. 208–215, and E.G.C.F. Atchley in *Trans. St Paul's Ecclesiol. Soc.,* Vol. IV (1896–1900), pp. 161–176). The *In principio* is the final portion of a Welsh charm (for a disease in horses) recorded in the *Welsh Leech Book* (p. 95, no. 561).
44 Pp. 135–152.
45 Pp. 133–4.
46 See n. 9.
47 Pp. 157 and 159–161.
48 Pp. 162–9.
49 P. 177.
50 Pp. 158 (a note on herbs) and 171 (two recipes).
51 Pp. 179–193.
52 Pp. 197–200.

53 Pp. 214-8. This is not the same regimen as the one given in B.M., fols. 16 *recto*-17 *verso* and M.M., pp. 62-8.

54 Pp. 228-237. A useful commentary on this famous work is to be found in Lynn Thorndike, *A History of Magic and Experimental Science*, Vol. II (1923), pp. 267-278, and *The Journal of the Royal Asiatic Society*, 1908, pp. 1065-1084 (M. Gaster, ' An Introduction to the Hebrew Version . . .') See also *ibid.:* pp. 111-162, for Gaster's translation of the Hebrew version, which he had published in the *Journal* for 1907.

55 Thorndike, *op. cit.*, pp. 269-70 ; Gaster, *art. cit.*, 1069-70. Philip translated the whole work, whereas John of Spain had been content to translate one book only (Book XII). Bened's Welsh version is based on John of Spain's translation.

56 B.M., fols. 48 *verso*-52 *verso*. It is also found in H., pp. 14-9.

57 One only is complete and bearing the author's name. It is a poem (pp. 208-10) by Ieuan Brydydd Hir (fl. *circa* 1450). I have succeeded in identifying two others as incomplete versions of poems by Llywelyn ap Gutun (pp. 204-6), a harpist and poet of the late fifteenth century, and Deio ab Ieuan Du (fl. 1460-80)—his elegy on the death of Rhys ap Maredudd of Tywyn, near Cardigan (pp. 238-41).

58 C. G. Kuhn (ed.) : *Claudii Galeni opera omnia* (Leipzig, 1826), Vol. XI.

59 *The Cyrurgie of Guy de Chauliac*, ed. M. S. Ogden (E. E. T. S., No. 265), 1971, pp. 616-631.

60 Warren Dawson : *Magician and Leech* (1929), pp. 141-7 ; *idem, A Leechbook of the XVth Century* (1934), pp. 12-16.

61 It is not impossible that ' Pyrrili ', whose opinion on the medicinal virtues of betony is referred to in Soth., p. 88, is a garbled form of Pliny's name.

62 Bened's manuscript, as we have seen (notes 8 and 42), contains a Christian charm.

63 They formulated the renowned *Regimen sanitatis Salernitanum*, which had a wide influence throughout the Middle Ages.

64 See n. 2.

65 See notes 27, 28 and 33.

66 Soth., pp. 64-5. *Cf* B.M., fols. 22 *verso*-23 *verso* ; M.M., pp. 28-32 ; H., pp. 70-71 ; Rawl., fol. 23 *recto*.

67 Soth., p. 93. *Cf* B.M., fols. 20 *recto*—21 *recto* ; M.M., pp. 8-10.

68 Soth., p. 80. *Cf* M.M., p. 120 ; H., p. 81 ; Rawl., fol. 26 *verso*.

69 Soth., pp. 79-80. *Cf* M.M., p.122 ; H., p. 96.

70 Soth., p. 47. *Cf* H., p. 21.

71 Soth., p. 56. *Cf* B.M., fols. 41 *verso*-42 *recto*.

72 Soth., p. 65. *Cf* H., p. 21 ; Rawl., fol 20 *verso*. See also Hens., p. 68.

73 Soth., pp. 73-4. *Cf* M.M., pp. 120-122 ; H., p. 97.

74 Soth., p. 77. *Cf* H., p. 36.

75 Soth., p. 87. *Cf* B.M., fol. 19 *recto* ; M.M., p. 40 ; Rawl., fol. 24 *recto*.

76 Soth., p. 87. *Cf* J., p. 140.

77 Soth., p. 94. *Cf* Rawl., fol. 21 *verso*.

78 Soth., p. 95. *Cf* M.M., p. 38 ; Rawl., fol. 23 *verso*.

79 Soth., p. 96. *Cf* M.M., p. 40.

80 Soth., p. 62. *Cf* J., p. 156.

81 Examples are : (1) An ointment (for an unspecified purpose)—Soth., p. 49. *Cf* B.M., fol. 36 *recto-verso*. (2) An ointment for a pain caused by a 'cold humour'—Soth., p. 50. *Cf* H., p. 83. (3) Another ointment for the same condition and for the palsy—Soth., pp. 50-51. *Cf* B.M., fols. 44 *verso*-45 *recto* ; H., p. 84. (4) An ointment (attributed to Hippocrates) for the palsy and for every kind of pain arising from a 'cold humour'—Soth., p. 51. *Cf* B.M., fol. 45 *recto* and *verso* ; H., p. 84. (5) An ointment (known as *Eli twf*) for promoting growth—Soth., p. 58. *Cf* B.M., fols. 38 *verso* and 47 *recto*.

82 Soth., pp. 49-50. *Cf* B.M., fols. 36 *verso*-38 *recto* ; H., pp. 40, 99. Bened records only the prologue, which enumerates the virtues of the remedy ; the recipe may not, perhaps, have been available to him.

83 Two remedies bearing the name *Gratia Dei* are to be found in a number of Middle English manuscripts—e.g., Hens., pp. 48-50, 53-4 ; Th., p. 68 ; Dawson, *Leechbook:* p. 118. Dr Ogden informs us (Th., p. 113) that Jean Pitard, a French Court surgeon in the fourteenth century, seems to have been the first writer to record an unguent of this name (see Karl Sudhoff's edition of Pitard's manual in *Archiv für Geschichte der Medizin*, II (1909), p. 213).

84 Th., p. 113 (note on 68.1-12), and the ref. cited therein.

85 His recipe for inducing wakefulness (p. 62) is found in Rawl., fols. 19 *verso*-20 *recto* as a prescription for promoting hair growth.

86 P. 42.

87 *The School of Salernum. Regimen sanitatis salernitanum,* trans. by Sir J. Harington, ed. F. Packard and F. H. Garrison, (London, 1922), pp. 124, 173. Fennel, vervain, rue and the rose are also prescribed, and it is interesting to note that fennel and rue are ingredients, in conjunction with the celandine, in three of Bened's other eye remedies (pp. 42-3). Fennel and celandine are included also in a recipe for an eye ointment in M.M., p. 142, and H., pp. 82, 61.

88 Tobit's sight was restored by fish gall (Book of *Tobit*, VI, 8-9 ; XI, 13). Pliny recommended the gall of a small animals, and the Arab physicians followed his example. Constantinus Africanus specifies the gall of a hare as a remedy for making the eyes clear. See Th., p. 88, note on a recipe (p. 11/28-32) which contains two of the gall ingredients found in Bened's recipe. The gall of a cockerel is found in many eye recipes, e.g., the Welsh recipe in M.M. and in H., cited in n. 87 *supra,* and an English recipe in Dawson, *Leechbook*, p. 164 (no. 496).

89 P. 42.

90 P. 58.

91 Th., p. 58. The editor has a valuable note on pp. 107-8.

92 It would seem, from a consideration of the kind of scribal errors which are to be found in Bened's book, that his sources were chiefly written, rather than oral. Examples are *erav* (for *crav*), p. 4, and *new* (for *neu*), p. 14, which seem clearly to be errors of the eye, rather than errors of the ear or the hand.

SOME HEALING AND HOLY WELLS OF WALES*

MARSHALL W. ANNEAR

I WATER, WELLS, AND AGENCIES OF HEALING

An important worldwide feature in religious and healing practice, has been the worship of water, particularly of its sources. Beliefs and practices in well-and spring-worship, have been shared by other cultures in other ages. To ancient Egyptians, the Nile was a god, and purifying water was used in healing. In ancient Greece, healing temples were built in groves near springs or streams, which were venerated, as were their ruling deities, with resultant legends and myths. Examples survive at Amphiarion and on Cos, home of Hippocrates. The pool of Bethesda at Jerusalem is famous, as are the Roman Baths at Bath. Offerings of precious stones and human sacrifices were made by the ancient Mayans of the Yucatan, at the sacred cenote, while the Inca of South America had his sacred bath for personal use. Even today, the Ganges is sacred in India, and an object of pilgrimage. In the British Isles and Eire, well-worship and legends are usually linked with a local saint, and such sites became important centres of healing in the past, in the same manner as can be seen in Ethiopia today at Debra Libanos. The present study refers to Wales, but early beliefs and practices express fundamental emotional needs.

To our ancestors, disease was ' unclean ', regarded as evil and linked with sin. Help came from religion (in Wales the Celtic Church) and from the purifying effects of water, particularly the water supply of the local saint. Sites of hermitages often had pre-Christian associations, but later acquired religious sanctity, and became centres of healing, particularly in the Middle Ages. After the Reformation, scepticism led to a decline in well-worship, but later, the supposed medicinal qualities of some wells, led to the development of spas. In recent

*—A *précis* of a paper profusely illustrated with slides.

times interest has moved to the myths and their significance in the psychology of social and cultural change.

II SOME OF THE HOLY AND HEALING WELLS OF WALES

Wales is rich in hallowed springs and wells associated with early Celtic saints who, with few material possessions, but rich in learning, were venerated as bringers of faith and hope of healing to those afflicted with sin or the Devil. Offerings of pins, coins, or tokens of recovery such as crutches were given at the well-shrine, as can be seen today in Eire, and once occurred at St Govans, Pembrokeshire. Sometimes well-localities were scenes of dancing on specific dates, while at some the performance of a difficult feat granted a wish. Patients at the out-patient clinics today, would formerly have gathered at well-shrines, as at Ffynnon Degla for the cure of St Tegla's Disease (Epilepsy) or at Ffynnon Taf at Taff's Well used from Roman times until the mid-nineteenth century, of which Mr and Mrs S. C. Hall gave a vivid description in 1861 in *The Book of South Wales, the Wye, and the Coast*. Today it is forgotten. Ffynnon Fair on Mynydd Penrhys was famous for cures in the early part of the sixteenth century. Although after the dissolution of the monasteries crowds were discouraged, its reputation persisted, and it has since been restored.

Breconshire has fewer well-shrines than Glamorgan, but with Radnorshire includes the area of the erstwhile famous spas of Llanwrtyd Wells, Llangammarch Wells, Builth Wells and Llandrindod Wells. Only at the last named is the medicinal water still available at the now deserted pump-room. Water still flows at Dolycoed, and the changing rooms still stand at Victoria Wells, Llanwrtyd, the pump-room at Llangammarch is almost hidden by trees while at Builth, Glannau Wells have all-but disappeared and Park Wells have been incorporated in a fine residence. Search among lanes east of Llandrindod Wells reveal a wooden cabin with a rusting pipe from which sulphurous water still flows, once used for the 'falling sickness' at Llandegla Well.

At Llanfechain, Montgomeryshire, Ffynnon Armon once covered by a stone structure, was used for total immersion in baptism and for bathing the sick, while further north at Holywell in Flintshire, Saint Winifred's Well still stands in its former glory, its fame being such that it escaped destruction at the dissolution of the monasteries. Cloaked in legend, dating from the seventh century, it was visited by the famous, including James II and his queen, praying to be blessed with a son. To this day it is visited by pilgrims, bathing and religious services being permitted at specific times.

In Denbighshire at Llanrhaeadr, is the rectangular ruin of Ffynnon Ddyfnog, believed to be effective for scabs and itch and even the pox, while near St Georges at Kinmel Park is Ffynnon Gegidog, capable of curing sick horses if they were sprinkled with its water, St Kegidog being the Celtic patron saint of horsemen.

Anglesey possesses numerous holy wells ; that of St Seiriol at Penmon still shows the ruined cell of the saint adjoining the baptismal well, which in recent times has been used as a wishing well for lovers. This sixth century saint was a friend of St Cybi and they met for their mid-day meal near Llanerchymedd, where each had a well. That of St Seiriol remains and was visited at night by the sick until mid-nineteenth century. On Holyhead Island close by Rhoscolyn, near to the cliff edge lies Ffynnon Wenfaen. St Gwenfaen had founded a religious cloister nearby. It was reputed to cure melancholy, while near the coast at Llaneilian is the well of St Eilian, which had a dual purpose, not only for healing ague, fits, scrofula and sore eyes, but also for divining the future and laying curses. On Llanddwyn Island once the home of St Dwynwen and now a Nature Reserve, are the remains of the church of St Dwynwen and her well. In the past it was visited by distressed lovers, praying for success or forgetfulness, a custom having its origin in the legend of St Dwynwen. She had a vision of being offered a goblet full of tranquilising liquid, when in distress concerning her lover Maelor. In later years, an old woman from Newborough was in attendance, to prognosticate the lovers' success from the movement of eels in the well.

Caernarvonshire is likewise rich in healing wells; one at a point of embarkation for Bardsey being Ffynnon Fair, below high-tide line at the foot of Mynydd Mawr, already mentioned regarding a wishing legend. Another is that of St Beuno near the church at Clynnog, where children with the ' falling sickness ' spent the night on a stone in the floor after being bathed in the well at eventide. It is still in a good state of preservation, as is the well of St Cybi at Llangybi, which in the mid-eighteenth century was embellished with a bath-house. The movements of an eel foretold the future ; also the lame, the halt and the blind frequented the site, or water was conveyed to them in bottles if they were too infirm. The lake at Glasfryn, adjoining

Ffynnon Grasi, is reputed to have been formed when a woman named Grace failed to close the door of the well-house, her home was submerged, and she became a swan on the lake until her death.

Pembrokeshire has many wells, several named after St David. The one in the Cathedral Churchyard is used to provide clean water for mass, while that dedicated to his mother, St Non stands near her ruined chapel by the shore and has recently been restored. St Non was also venerated in Cornwall, where at Alternun near Launceston, under a thorn bush, is all that remains of her well. This was used for those mentally disordered or ' possessed ', who were tumbled in the waters in a process known as ' bowesening ' or ducking, and thereafter conveyed to the church for masses to be sung over them. The deserted and ruined St Edrin's church (Pembrokeshire) once had a churchyard well with a reputation for curing madness. It dried up when used for washing clothes on a Sunday, and its powers were transferred to the churchyard grass, which is reputed to preserve men and cattle from the bite of a mad dog. Similar powers of curing madness were attributed to a well and the surrounding grass in the ' Valley of the Mad ' in Eire. St Govans Well in south Pembrokeshire, already mentioned, was for the cure of ' diverse illnesses ' or ' many distempers '.

Many interesting wells lie within Carmarthenshire, one near Pendine (Ffynnon Nathan) having spa reputation. That of St Anthony at Llansteffan was once of repute as a healing well, but now is regarded as a ' wishing well '.

The study of healing shrines in early times in Wales would be incomplete without reference to the legend of the Physicians of Myddfai. The first of that name practised their art in the early years of the thirteenth century, but according to legend, they were originally the sons of the Lady of Llyn y Fan Fach. A local shepherd saw her sitting on an island in the lake, courted her and married her. Her terms were that she would return to the lake if he ever struck her three careless blows. They lived happily for many years having three sons to whom she imparted medical lore. Alas, her husband struck her carelessly three times and she returned to the lake with all her cattle. The symbolic significance of this legend raises many questions, including the possibility of folk memory.

III SUMMARY AND CONCLUDING OBSERVATIONS

A brief outline of beliefs of earlier peoples in other parts of the world provided a background for the subject of the beliefs and customs related to the holy and healing wells of Wales. There is no clear distinction between wells-holy, and wells-healing, as in earlier ages they were almost synonymous. The associated legends frequently have border-line medical interest.

Finally, attention must be drawn to the importance of water in the context of the human psyche. A pre-1939 picture by Brierly Russell entitled *The Lost Generation* was enigmatic, until it was realised that it attempted to depict the symbolism of the healing aspect of water as expressed in the last chapter of the *Book of the Revelation* (verses 1-8), 'And he showed me a pure river of water of life . . . In the midst of it . . . was there the Tree of Life . . . and the leaves of the tree were for the healing of the nations'. This expresses the universal healing aspect of water, linked with our concepts of the divine and holy, as we have seen expressed in our wanderings among the Holy and Healing Wells of Wales.

ACKNOWLEDGEMENT

The author wishes to record his gratitude to Major Francis Jones, Wales Herald of Arms Extraordinary for the inspiration given by his book *The Holy Wells of Wales* (1954).

JOHN COAKLEY LETTSOM'S WELSH CONNEXIONS

D. Geraint James

During May 1973 we celebrated the bicentenary of the Medical Society of London, founded by John Coakley Lettsom (1744-1815) (James 1973).

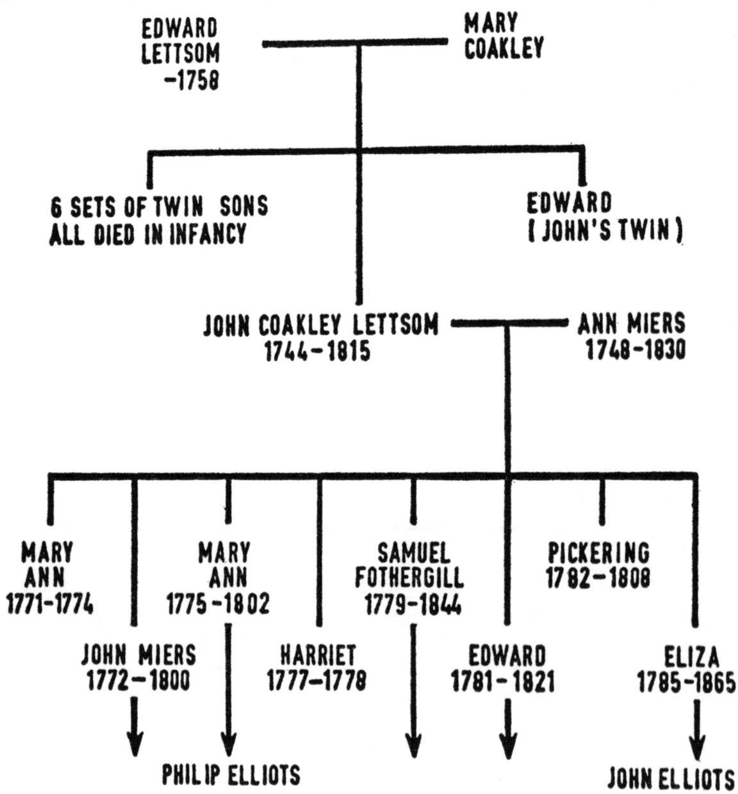

Figure 1. The Lettsom Family Tree

He was born in Tortola, Virgin Islands, son of Edward Lettsom and Mary Coakley (Fig. 1). He and his brother Edward were the only surviving twins of seven sets of twins, all the others having died in infancy (Johnston Abraham 1933). His descendants, spanning the 18th and 19th centuries, are numerous and interesting (Fig. 1). What appeals particularly to Welsh historians are his Welsh connexions.

FAMILY PORTRAIT

The Wellcome Institute of the History of Medicine exhibits a charming portrayal of Lettsom with his wife, Ann Miers, & their family in the garden of their home at Grove Hill, Camberwell. (Plate 13). Mother Ann Miers Lettsom sits at the far left of the painting and at her left are successively Mary Ann Lettsom (Mrs Philip Elliot) and Eliza (Mrs John Elliot) ; Pickering Lettsom is clutching the dog. Father's right hand is resting on the left shoulder of John Miers Lettsom and his hand is entwined in that of Samuel Fothergill Lettsom.

The original oils on canvas, 69 x 79 cm, is ascribed to John Zoffany (1734/5-1810). Art experts question this and instead attribute it to a pupil of Arthur Devis (1708-1787) (F. N. L. Poynter, personal communication). The painting has been in the possession of John Hugh Armstrong Elliot, great-great-grandson of Lettsom through John Elliot. The Wellcome bought the painting in 1917 from Puttick and Simpson's.

Lettsom had eight children, four sons and four daughters. This family portrait does not include two daughters, Mary Ann and Harriet,

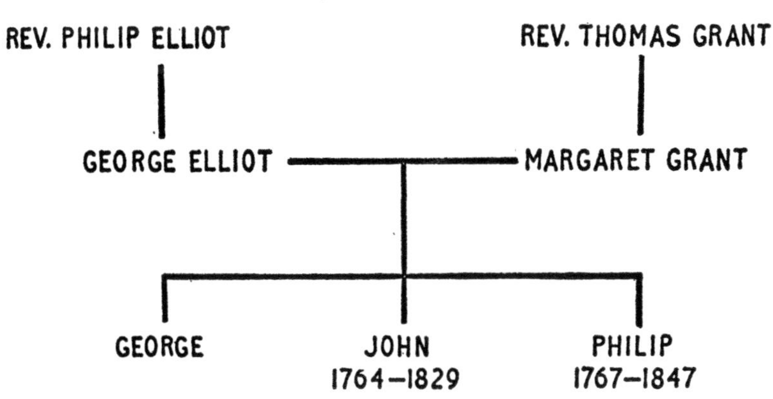

Figure 2. The Elliot Family Tree

both of whom died in infancy, nor does it include Edward (1781-1821) a hydrocephalic epileptic imbecile.

LAUGHARNE, NEATH AND SWANSEA

Two Lettsom daughters married two brothers, Philip and John Elliot, who came from an old established Welsh Pembrokeshire family. George Elliot of St Botolph's, the sixth son of the Rev. Philip Elliot, married Margaret, daughter of the Rev. Thomas Grant, Rector of Nolton (Fig. 2) (Johnston Abraham, 1933). George became a surgeon in Laugharne, Carmarthenshire, where his three sons—George, John (1764-1829) and Philip (1767-1847) were born. There were also Welsh connexions on the maternal side, because a John Grant owned and lived in Gnoll Castle, Neath, and bore his coat of arms there. A descendant of this family, Dr Alan Grant, is a Belfast Consulting Physician, who will undoubtedly one day set out in print his distinguished ancestry.

Philip Elliot (1767-1847) left Laugharne to do medicine at Edinburgh where he qualified M.D. on June 24th 1791, spent a little time at St Mary's Hall, Oxford, and then started to practise medicine at Swansea. He had scarcely settled into practice when he met Mary Ann Lettsom (1775-1802) who came to stay at Gnoll Castle, Neath, on a visit to her cousin, Lady Mackworth. Lady Mackworth was not only a close friend and counsellor but also a near relation, for she was a Miers, the wealthy and distinguished Quaker family into which John Coakley Lettsom had married on July 31st, 1770.

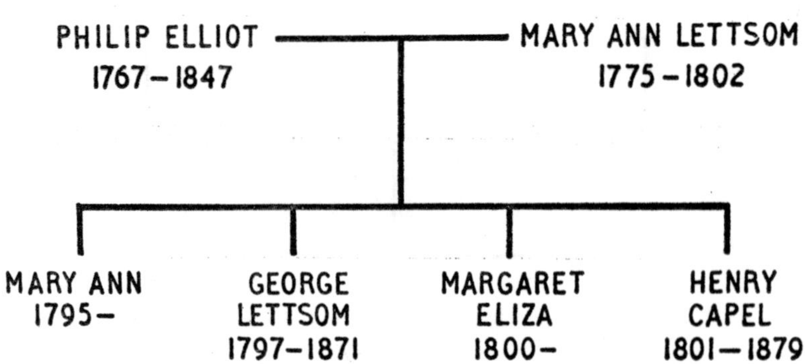

Figure 3. Dr Philip Elliot's Family

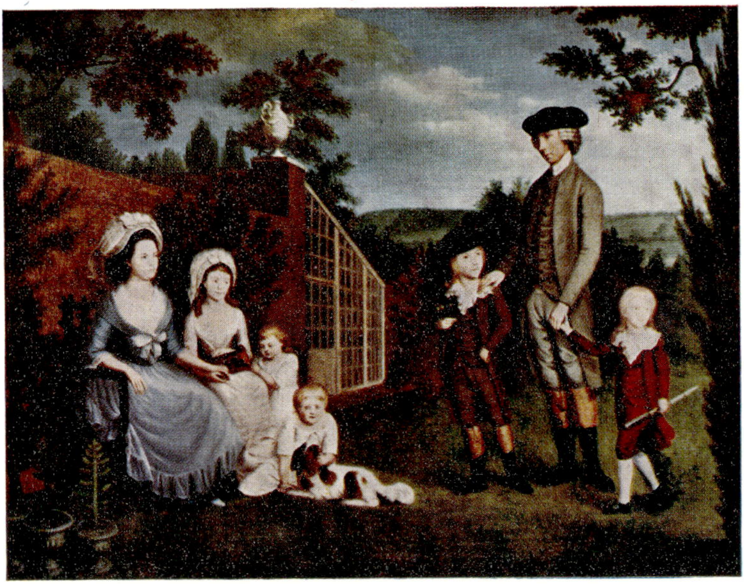

Plate 13
John Coakley Lettsom and his family at Grove Hill, Camberwell.
Attributed to John Zoffany.
(By kind permission of the Wellcome Trustees).

and Reid, and now Watney Mann Ltd. Here then is a direct link from John Coakley Lettsom through the Welsh Elliots to Red Barrel beer and, through Maxwell Joseph's Grand Metropolitan Hotels' Group to the Express Dairy Milk Chain. John Coakley Lettsom, the teetotal Quaker, would undoubtedly have approved of this link in the chain.

THE GLAMORGANSHIRE TINPLATE WORKS

When John Miers died in 1787 he directed that his nephews, John Nathaniel Miers and Samuel Fothergill Lettsom, should have the option of taking over his family tinplate works in Glamorgan (Abraham 1933). The two cousins took over and maintained the family name John Miers and Co. until about 1810 when their diverging policies caused a split. The expansive Samuel Fothergill Lettsom retained the name of John Miers and Co. for his works at Ynysygerwn, Dulais and Avon, and also drew his father-in-law Sir William Garrow into the business. However, his was a Welsh disaster, for he went bankrupt at the expense of his manager, Vigurs, who amassed a fortune from this enterprise (Brooks 1932). Samuel Fothergill Lettsom died in bankruptcy in 1844 in Boulogne and his wife died in 1857 and was buried at Christ Church, Folkestone (Fig. 4).

His cousin, John Nathaniel Miers, took over the Ynyspenllwch works, trading under the name J. N. Miers and Co. successfully until his death in 1814.

NAME	BORN	DIED	BURIED
Edward Lettsom		1758	Tortola
John Coakley L.	1744	1815	Bunhill Fields
Ann Miers L.	1748	1830	Bunhill Fields
John Miers L.	1772	1800	Bunhill Fields
Mrs Philip Elliot	1767	1847	Bunhill Fields
William Nanson L.	1796	1865	Paddington
Louisa L.	1799	1866	Paddington
Mary Ann L.	1797	1832	Torquay
Samuel Fothergill L.	1779	1844	Boulogne
Eliza Sophia L.	1784	1857	Folkestone
Pickering L.	1782	1808	Tortola
Ruth L.		1809	Tortola
John Elliot	1764	1829	St Mgts. Westminster
Mrs John Elliot	1785	1865	Brompton

Figure 4. Burial Grounds of members of the Lettsom family

SUMMARY

The large and remarkable Lettsom and Miers families were closely intertwined in many different fashions with Wales.

Two Welsh-born Carmarthenshire brothers married two Lettsom sisters. One brother practised medicine in Swansea and the other maintained a London Welsh Open Arms-style home in Pimlico for his many Welsh relations.

The Miers side of the family owned tinplate works in Glamorganshire. Some of these prospered, others failed, but all undoubtedly contributed to the versatility of this truly remarkable and exciting family of Friends.

This contribution to the first ever Welsh Congress on the History of Medicine serves to remind us of their Welshness.

REFERENCES

Abraham, J. J. (1933). *Lettsom*. Heinemann, London.
Brooke, E. H. (1932). *Monograph on the Tinplate works in Great Britain.* Welsh Plate and Steel Manufacturers' Association, Swansea.
James, D. G. (1973). *New Engl. J, Med.,* 288, 1124.
Janes, Hurford (1963). *The Red Barrel.* Murray, London.

DR THOMAS WILLIAMS OF SWANSEA, 1818-65[1]

PETER H. THOMAS

Thomas Williams, the outstanding physician and scientist, was one of many children belonging to the Reverend John Williams, vicar of Llandyfrïog, Cardiganshire. Extremely studious in youth, Thomas Williams had very little to help him in his progress beyond good example and good advice—the rest that was necessary came from within himself. Having been apprenticed to a certain Mr Terry until he was about nineteen years of age, he enrolled in 1837 as a medical student at Guy's Hospital where he soon revealed his remarkable talents and strength of character. As an undergraduate he published some short papers in the *Medical Gazette,* gained several prizes and, at the Physical Society, was given some of his initial experience in scientific debate. Even at this stage of his career he evinced unmistakeable proof of his intellectual ability. In 1839 he qualified as a M.R.C.S. (England) and, in the following year he successfully sat his M.B. (London) ; he was, therefore, one of the earliest graduates in medicine from that university. In 1841 his original botanical paper entitled ' On the structure and uses of the stomata ' appeared in the *Microscopical Journal.*[2] Two years later, when scarcely twenty-four years old, he won the Triennial Prize of fifty guineas presented by the Royal College of Surgeons (England), for an essay describing the results of his investigations on ' The structure and functions of the lungs '.

Having quickly grasped the cell-doctrine of Schwann, Williams used the achromatic microscope—an instrument perfected by J. J. Lister in 1830—to undertake original research in the field of microbiology and histo-pathology. This Welshman was one of the first investigators at Guy's to have understood the full significance of the microscope. He realised at once how the new optical aid would not only revolutionise scientific thought and attitudes but also clinical teaching. He advocated that Lister's improved instrument should be accepted universally as the inseparable tool of the morbid anatomist. Early in his career, Williams filled the office of demonstrator in (microscopic) structural anatomy and curator of the microscopic department at Guy's, but seeing no opening for promotion, he joined the privately-owned Webb Street School[3] as teacher of anatomy and lectured for a short period on forensic medicine. At the school on 14th February, 1843 the Welsh doctor was invited to dissect the body of the political extremist, Richard Carlile.

In 1843, the Welsh doctor contributed an article 'On the pathology of cells' to *Guy's Hospital Reports* in which he reviewed the work done on cellular pathology, starting with the pioneering observations of Johannes Müller, Grüby, Raspail, Rokitansky, Bowman, Addison, and Wharton Jones. Among other outstanding investigators mentioned by Williams in the *Report* were Purkinje, Henle, R.de Graaf, Liebig, John Hunter, Cullen, Magendie, Owen Rees, Richard Owen, Kuhn, and Cruveilhier. The main part of the article, supported by references to relevant English and continental literature, consisted of a discussion of the microscopic changes which took place in cells and tissues in inflammation, liver degeneration, and cancer, with possible causes for these conditions. A feature of the *Report* and, indeed, of his later writings, was that he never refrained from being scathingly critical when the occasion demanded it—perhaps, too critical, for his slender years. His second contribution to *Guy's Hospital Reports* entitled 'On the physiology of cells, with a view to elucidate the laws regulating the structure and function of the glands', appeared in 1846. His third and last contribution in this publication, entitled 'On the physical conditions affecting the distribution of life in the sea and the atmosphere and the laws of acquatic breathing', appeared two years later.

Attainments, ability, a flair for languages, the opinions of his contemporaries, all marked Dr Williams as a man whose proper sphere was a consultancy at a London teaching hospital. There was, unfortunately, no likely vacancy for any higher position than tutor at Guy's and his health was not robust. At an early period of his life he developed renal dropsy from which he made an apparent recovery and which prompted him to record the details of his case in one of the medical journals. Not long after the closure of the Webb Street School in 1843, he settled down for the rest of his life in Wind Street, Swansea, where he commenced private practice, and later, became physician to the old Infirmary situated in Paxton Street.[4] It must be realised that when he returned to Wales, Williams brought with him all the skill, information, and opinions of a first-rate London man. He was the type of individual who was never satisfied unless he maintained his professional learning at the highest level. He was constantly buying new books, he subscribed to numerous medical and scientific journals, and was in receipt of many foreign publications. Every new device in the way of a medical or surgical instrument became part of his equipment because he knew that such a device would facilitate diagnosis and afford better treatment for his patients. In 1845, he proceeded to the degree of M.D., London University.

Although Dr Williams devoted the major portion of his time to the conduct of an ever-increasing practice, the remainder was given over to literary and scientific pursuits. In 1844 he published an interesting book entitled *A sketch of the relation which subsists between the three kingdoms of nature : mineral, vegetable, and animal . . .* The work was dedicated to Lewis Weston Dillwyn, F.R.S., F.G.S., President of the Royal Institution of South Wales. Shortly after his arrival in Swansea Williams became a member of that learned body where he continued to play an extremely important and active part throughout the rest of his life. The purpose of the publication was to try to popularise science among the townsfolk who, at that time, according to him, showed a decided lack of interest in the educational facilities afforded by the Royal Institution. He served for many years as honorary curator in the Institution's department of entomology and later acted in a similar capacity in the department of zoology until his death.

Evidently, the Welsh doctor excelled in the inter-related subjects of physiology, zoology, and comparative anatomy. As a marine biologist he revelled in the wealth of strange and wonderful creatures which were plentiful in the sea around the coasts of Swansea Bay and the Gower Peninsula. In order to obtain live specimens for his research he even employed special dredges which were operated from boats provided with winches for reeling in line. An accomplished draughtsman, he drew accurate elaborate sketches of what he revealed in his countless dissections in order to explain, illustrate, and permanently record the results of his investigations for the benefit of future workers in the same field of inquiry.

Dr Williams played an active part in the eighteenth annual meeting of the British Association for the Advancement of Science which was held at Swansea from 9-16 August 1848 under the presidency of the

Marquess of Northampton. The fact that the event awakened a genuine interest in science among the ordinary local townsfolk was very important to people like Williams who were constantly striving to stimulate some general enthusiasm for natural philosophy through the medium of lectures, experiments, and demonstrations at the Royal Institution. Summaries of two of Williams' zoological papers were published in the *British Association Reports* for that year. In the same organ, three years later, he published his 'Report on the British annelida ', a work which bore the stamp of such intensive research and frequently referred to in Professor Rymer Jones' standard book entitled *An outline of the organisation of the animal kingdom*. In addition, he wrote an item in the *Reports* entitled ' On the structure of the branchiae and mechanism of breathing in the Pholades and other lamelli branchiate molluscs '.

The twenty-first anniversary meeting[5] of the Provincial Medical and Surgical Association (two years later to become the British Medical Association) was held at Swansea on 10 and 11 August, 1853 under the Presidency of Dr Gwynne Bird, a practitioner of the town. At that gathering Dr Williams communicated two papers, the first of which, entitled ' Origin, transformation, and decline of the floating cells of the blood ', was illustrated by many instructive diagrams. The second communication bearing the title ' Ultimate structure of the air-cells considered in its relation to certain of their diseases ' consisted of a brief explanation of drawings relevant to the subject under discussion. The convention at Swansea also afforded a splendid opportunity for provincial physicians like Williams to meet under the chairmanship of Charles Hastings to discuss a report on the newly-proposed Charter of the Royal College of Physicians, London. It is noteworthy that the Welsh doctor was an Extra-Licentiate of the College.

There were no limits to Williams' scientific endeavors. Viewed against the pressure of his day-to-day work as a doctor, his intellectual activity was all the more remarkable. In 1853 he published a tripartite series entitled ' The blood : its chemistry, physiology and pathology ' in the *British and Foreign Medico-Chirurgical Review*. From 1853-7 inclusively his illustrated series ' On the mechanism of aquatic respiration and on the structure of the organs of breathing in invertebrate animals appeared by instalments in the *Annals of Natural History*. In 1857 the whole series ' On the mechanism of aquatic respiration . . .'

with the subtitle 'The structure, functions, and diseases of the lungs' was reprinted for convenience under one cover to form a monograph. The monograph, according to Williams, represented only one part of a wider study which he was making of respiration and lung disorders. The additional work was never published but in the same year, however, he contributed an article on the 'Structure of the lungs of man and the vertebrate animals' to Todd's *Cyclopaedia.*

In 1852 Williams' first paper, 'On the blood proper and chylaqueous fluid of invertebrate animals' appeared in the *Philosophical Transactions.* His second paper, 'Researches on the structure and homology of the reproductive organs of the annelids' was published in the same journal six years later. The inclusion of a paper in the Transactions of the Royal Society was itself a sufficient guarantee of merit since all scientific manuscripts underwent the most careful scrutiny before publication was even considered. The amount of labour involved in the two investigations can only be appreciated by reference to the papers themselves which are copiously illustrated. For these and numerous other original contributions to medical and scientific literature he was elected a Fellow of the Royal Society on 3 June 1858. It is interesting to note that since 1848 the honour of admission to the Society has been jealously guarded. His election to the Fellowship of the Linnean Society[6] took place on 17 April 1855.

For students of medical and social history Williams' *Report on the copper smoke, its influence on the public health, and the industrial diseases of coppermen* (Swansea, 1854) is a very important publication. In the first part of the *Report* he gave an elaborate account of an environmental study which he had made of the twelve thousand local copper men and colliers inhabiting a district measuring ten by three miles. He remarked that the copper-smelting industry had given to Swansea an international reputation, to its merchants opulence, and to its artisans abundance. The success of the trade was due to the immediate proximity of the smelting-works to the extensive collieries in the neighbourhood. Williams stated that the surface of the land to the north and north-east of Swansea looked as if it were scorched. The region was practically denuded of vegetation as a direct result of the action of the sulphurous copper smoke which, in fifteen decades of smelting operations, had transformed the smiling valley into a barren desert.

In the second part of the *Report* Dr Williams gave an account of the

Great Copper Trial[7]—the name given to the celebrated lawsuit heard at Carmarthen in 1833. In the indictment preferred against Messrs Vivian, owners of the Hafod Works, Swansea, it was alleged that the copper smoke from their furnaces was injurious to animal life and destructive to vegetation. Farm animals eating grass soured by sulphurous fumes from the copper smoke became afflicted with a disease locally known as *effryddod*. At the end of the trial a verdict was returned in favour of the defendants. The lawsuit had failed because the industry was considered to be so important to the wealth of Swansea and district. The coppermasters had won the day !

Even at the age of forty-six Williams was still an eligible bachelor. He had travelled widely in Europe. Although he had accomplished much in the fields of medicine and biology, his research programme was far from complete. He was, however, not totally oblivious to the charms of the fair sex because on 25 January 1865 he married Eliza Dennis, second daughter of the late Dr Archibald C. Ross, M.D., Madeira. Only a few months later he was taken suddenly ill at his home in Wind Street, Swansea. The illness, which proved to be fatal, was agonisingly painful though mercifully short. Having been married for four brief months, with every prospect of future happiness, the distinguished physician and scientist passed away on 23 May 1865 at his own residence. During the twenty or more years that Dr Williams had served the people of the Swansea area, he was respected for his high principles, his earnest dedication to his profession, and the humane manner in which he treated his patients. From 1845 onwards he worked unceasingly for the good of the Royal Institution of South Wales. A superb lecturer[8] and teacher, he did everything within his grasp to promote the various scientific and literary aims of that establishment. He was an ardent Welshman, steeped in the antiquities and literature of his native land. He had studied language with as much passion as he had devoted to comparative anatomy and medicine. By sheer force of industry and talent Dr Williams had, within a comparatively short life-span, not only attained an unrivalled position in the Principality as a man of science and as a medical practitioner, but was widely recognised internationally.

REFERENCES

1 An augmented account of his life will be found in Williams, Stewart (ed.), *Glamorgan Historian*, Barry (Glam.), n.d. [1973], Vol. 9, pp. 70-95.
2 1841, 1, 118-121.
3 See Sir Zachary Cope's article "The private medical schools of London (1746-1914)" in Poynter, F.N.L. (ed.), *The Evolution of Medical Education in Britain*, Pitman, London, 1966, p. 97.
4 See illustrated article by E. Jenkins and C. Rogers, "Old photographs of Swansea", in Williams, Stewart (ed.), *Glamorgan Historian*, D. Brown, Cowbridge, 1965, Vol. 2.
5 For a full account of the meeting consult *Ass. med. J.*, 1853, 726-743,
6 Thomas Williams had read a ' book on the grave of Linnaeus, in the far north, by the silvery light almost of the midnight sun '. Quoted from his work entitled, *The Present Geographical Movement and Future Geographical Distribution of the English Race of Men*, Swansea, 1859.
7 *The Cambrian* newspaper dated 16 March, 1833, gives full and accurate coverage of the case.
8 For a list of his lectures, etc., see *Rep. R. Inst. S. Wales.*

FURTHER GENERAL REFERENCES

The primary sources from which biographical information has been obtained are the obituary notices in the Swansea newspaper *The Cambrian* (2 June, 1865), the *Lancet* (1, 637, 10 June, 1865, signed R. B.), and the *Dictionary of Welsh Biography*, ed. by J. E. Lloyd and R. T. Jenkins, (Hon. Soc. Cymmrodorion, London, 1959) ; S. Wilks and G. T. Bettany, *A biographical history of Guy's Hospital*, p. 428 (Ward, Lock, London, 1892) ; T. I. Jones, "The contributions of Welshmen to science" in *Trans. Soc. Cymmr.* (session 1932-3) ; and the *Ceithio Ms.* deposited at the National Library of Wales, Aberystwyth.

Material relating to the biological aspects of the work has been drawn from W. B. Cannon, *The way of an investigator* (Hafner, N. Y. and London, 1968) ; J. Barrett and C. M. Younge, *Collins pocket guide to the sea shore* (Collins, London, 1967) ; H. Mellanby, *Animal life in fresh water* (Methuen, London, 1938) ; A. E. Vines and N. Rees, *Plant and animal biology:* 3rd ed. (2 vols., Pitman, London, 1968) ; I. Asimov, *A Short history of biology* (Nelson, London, 1965) ; F. J. Cole, *A history of comparative anatomy* (Macmillan, London, 1944) ; and relevant articles in *Encyclopaedia Britannica*.

With regard to general medical matters, we have made frequent recourse to D. Guthrie, *A history of medicine* (Nelson, London, 1945) ; F. H. Garrison *An introduction to the history of medicine:* 4th ed. (Saunders, Philadelphia and London, 1929) ; and B. J. Stern, *Society and medical progress* (Oxford University Press, London, 1941).

SIR THOMAS LEWIS (1881-1945)

ARTHUR HOLLMAN

I had the immense good fortune to be a clerk on Sir Thomas Lewis's firm at University College Hospital in 1943 when his superb clinical instruction and very fine lectures quickly made their impact on the raw student, as did his gentleness in guiding the novice into proper methods of work—with no trace of superiority, sarcasm at one's gaucherie, or aggressiveness towards the ignorant. Moreover, we enjoyed seeing him at our Saturday night dances in the Medical School, even though we (and clearly his own consultant colleagues too) stood in awe of him at all times. My own short acquaintance with Lewis gives me no authority to speak personally of his life and work, so this paper relies chiefly on the writing of others whose works are detailed in the bibliography. However, I did have sense enough on the tenth anniversary of his death to ask several of his former pupils to write about him in an issue of the *U.C.H. Magazine* and this included a delightful contribution by the late Dr Paul D. White of Boston.

Thomas Lewis was born at Teigil House, Roath, Cardiff on 26th December, 1881. His mother, Catherine Hannah, was of Welsh-Somerset descent and his father, Henry, came from an old Welsh family of Monmouthshire yeomen whose arms were those of 1) Rhys Goch, 2) Howell of Caerleon, 3) Caradwg Freich Fras and 4) Howell Dola. Henry was a mining engineer and colliery owner who won the Albert Medal for bravery during rescue work underground. He was a widely read man with a library of several thousand volumes and although Lewis later attributed his success as a student largely to his father's stimulus and encouragement, he spent every spare moment in the fields and woods of Wales, something not difficult say his biographers for a determined youth who was educated almost entirely at home by his mother and a tutor.

This great love of the countryside never left him and is reflected in his desire to be buried in Llangasty Churchyard, Breconshire, overlooking Llangorse Lake, where from his boyhood ' he had gone again and again to be with wild creatures '. Before his 'teens, he had decided to take up medicine because he hoped that by becoming a doctor he might emulate the sleight of hand of the family physician who was an expert conjurer ! After passing the London matriculation at his second attempt he took up pre-clinical work in Cardiff where he was especially stimulated by the physiologist Swale Vincent : during this time he wrote the standard papers on the haemolymph glands. Then in 1902 he entered U.C.H., his medical home for the rest of his life. The entrance was by award of an exhibition and this is interesting because neither then nor later did he rely on his father's wealth to pursue his career. His University Gold Medal in 1905 with triple distinction in the M.B., B.S. was the prelude to a life full of honours, none more significant than the Copley Medal of the Royal Society (1941), previously awarded to only one clinician—Lord Lister. I just cannot understand how the Nobel Prize Committee failed in later years to give him that final accolade which he so much deserved. His subsequent forty years of research in physiology and medicine were preeminent by any standards.

Now for a few words about his introduction to cardiac physiology and cardiology. The precise details are not clear but in general it is obvious that during his two years as houseman to Victor Horsley and Thomas Barlow, he was meeting men of ability like Dale, Elliott, Starling, Bayliss and Cushny—often over lunch at the former ABC teashop in Tottenham Court Road. Leonard Hill gave him the impetus to work on the pulse and Lewis's first cardiological paper published on 15th September, 1908, in the *B.M.J.* was on, ' The pulse in aortic disease ; the relation of pulse curves to blood pressure '.

The work was continued in Starling's laboratory and naturally led to his meeting James Mackenzie (in 1908), who urged him to undertake an analysis of the irregular action of the heart. This was the take-off point for him and like a jet aircraft he soared with enormous energy far above contemporary work. The engine, to continue the simile, was Einthoven's string galvanometer which he bought with the help of a Beit Memorial Fellowship and there was a memorable meeting of the Royal Society of Medicine at U.C.H. on 20th March, 1912, when W. Einthoven and himself read papers on the ' Observations of the movements of the heart by means of electrocardiograms '. In the previous year, he had published the first edition of his famous book *The Mechanism of the Heart Beat,* which became the bible of electrocardiography and attracted young men the world over to study with him. Among the first, in 1913 was Paul White of Boston who later wrote, 'I reported to Dr Thomas Lewis for work. He stopped for a brief moment to greet me, as he stood in his cutaway morning coat at the operating table in his laboratory, massaging the heart of a dog with one hand whilst the other hand held his top hat and dress gloves before attending some official luncheon'. White went on to say that it took three months before he was barely spoken to again but that Lewis then suddenly asked him to join in the experimental work 'and from that moment my life in London changed to one of intensive research day and night . . . I instructed Lewis in the use of the slide rule and this clinched my position as a devoted slave of the master'. Lewis was then only thirty-two years old. His work from 1908 to 1925 gave him a complete mastery of all aspects of the electrophysiology of the heart and clinical disorders of the heartbeat, and led to his election as F.R.S. in 1918.

Having written in some detail about his early years, one now has, unfortunately to condense what would otherwise be a very long account of his later work. This is unavoidable when it is remembered that he wrote 229 scientific papers and twelve books or monographs (one going into six editions).

His work on the electrocardiogram, including his famous and lasting hypothesis of a 'circus movement' as the cause of atrial flutter and fibrillation, was interrupted by World War I. He was about to take charge of a Welsh Military Hospital in Mesopotamia (where his former chief, Horsley, died on active service) when the Medical Research Committee (later Council) invited him to investigate the condition known as 'soldier's heart'. He did this at the Military Heart Hospital with Allbutt, Mackenzie and Osler and the study was reported in his book, *The soldier's heart and the effort syndrome.* In 1921, he was knighted for his war work. By 1925, he had tired of elaborate electrocardiographic work and returned to his observations on the cutaneous vessels which he had started during the war. He was influenced also by a growing belief that man, not animals, was the correct subject for hospital based research. The notable feature of his experiments on the vascular reaction of the skin to injury was that they were carried out with the simplest apparatus and yet they led to another classical monograph, *The blood vessels of the human skin and their responses* (1927).

Much of his research work had been published in the journal *Heart* which, with the help of his friend Mackenzie, he had founded in 1909. Since the war years, his cardiac department at U.C.H. had been funded by the Medical Research Council. But now came a most important turning point of his life. He was aware of the doubt of other scientists and clinicians that clinical medicine was susceptible to the discipline of science, and he strongly contested the view that advances in medicine in the future would come chiefly from basic science laboratories and animal experiment. As a result of these deliberations, he became a crusader for the concept and discipline of 'Clinical Science'. In 1930, he re-named his department 'The Department of Clinical Research' and in 1933, changed the title of *Heart* to *Clinical Science.*

Lewis's third and last period of major research effort was concerned with his work on pain. Carried on for several years with his collaborators, Pickering, Kellgren and Pochin, it culminated in his 1942 monograph *Pain.* It lacks the sparkle of his earlier writings and one suspects that this subjective phenomenon taxed even his unique research talents to the utmost. Nevertheless, much was accomplished and the separateness of superficial and deep pain was emphasized.

Then a world war again changed his path and in 1941 he took over from Max Rosenheim—when Max joined the Army—the charge of U.C.H. clinical students who were then evacuated to Llandough Hospital. However, he continued to write and his last paper in 1945 on congenital tricuspid stenosis takes us back to that meeting with Einthoven in 1912 when they discussed the E.C.G. findings in congenital pulmonary stenosis. During his time at Llandough, he wrote a little known paper on Caleb Hillier Parry, 'A great Welsh Physician and Scientist'.

Finally, a note on his life. At the age of thirty-six he married Lorna Treharne James of Merthyr Tydfil. They had two daughters, one of whom lived with Dr and Mrs Paul White during the war, and a son, Christopher, who is a physician in Vancouver.

Lady Lewis did much to help her husband through his later career, interrupted as it was by serious illness. He had his first coronary thrombosis in 1927 and having it is said only slender knowledge of the disease, he was made to realise its significance by only the insistence of Dr H. M. Marvin of Yale, then a post-graduate student with him.

A second attack followed eight years later and he said to Sir Arthur Keith, ' Another arrow from the same quiver, my friend—and one of them will get me in the end '. He died on 17th March, 1945, after the fourth attack. I understand that he gave up cigarette smoking after his first attack and in his famous textbook on *Diseases of the Heart* (1933) he says, ' it were best that cardiac patients did not smoke at all ', and in characteristic scientific manner added, ' We may not know definitely that long continued smoking is injurious to the blood-vessels, but we have reason strongly to suspect it. '

He worked continuously for ten months of every year and grudged the time ' wasted ' by his department at weekends and on public holidays. So intense was his concentration on the task in hand that he even discouraged light conversation at lunch times in the medical school. The other two months were spent, at any rate before his later years, on an equally intensive study of ornithology. He was an expert cameraman who took superb photographs of birds, which he was proud to show visitors at Sunday tea times.

Many of the figures in his works he prepared himself—both photographs and drawings. And with Henry Dale, he produced and directed the 1928 film of Harvey's work on the circulation.

Let us hope that one day a full length biography of this extraordinary man will be written—though the task will be as formidable to the writer as Lewis's achievements have been to the world.

This man was a legend during his lifetime so what more can one say of him after his death ? One thing—his work and his influence endure.

BIBLIOGRAPHY

1 *Obituary Notices of Fellows of the Royal Society of London* 5, (1945), 179-202.
2 *American Heart Journal* 29, (1945), 419-420.
3 *British Medical Journal* 1, (1945), 461-463.
4 *Lancet* 1, (1945), 419-420.
5 *British Heart Journal* 8, (1946), 1-3.
6 *University College Hospital Magazine* 40, (1955), 63-74.

TWO COLLIERY DOCTORS
THE BROTHERS ARMSTRONG OF TREORCHY

A. D. Morris

My object in studying Medicine (and May God prosper it) is not to gain a name, but to do good to my fellow creatures and assist them in their hour of need. (Frank Buckland)

'How green was my valley then' was not descriptive of the valley of the Rhondda in the last decades of the nineteenth century, when 'J. R. Armstrong, M.D. Surgeon', put up his brass plate at the entrance to Aeron Villa in the little mining town of Treorchy, Rhondda. By the turn of the century the valley was not an attractive residential township, for it had lost its pristine greenness, and was one of the wettest places in the British Isles. The mountains once covered with luxuriant forests were now replaced with ugly mounds of slag, the ubiquitous tips. The valley had but one industry, coal mining, and coal-dust had penetrated everywhere.

John Richardson Armstrong was the third child of eleven children, and Fergus Armstrong was the youngest. John was born on April 19th 1872, and Fergus on December 9th 1887 at a farm in the parish of Llanfair Talhaearn, Denbighshire. Their father, Charles Armstrong, a Scotsman, had migrated from Scotland to north Wales where he took over a hill farm of five hundred acres. His son John was educated at a grammar school in St Asaph, and in 1888 he passed the Edinburgh University medical preliminary examination which admitted him to the university medical school. Four years later, in 1892, he graduated with the degrees of M.B. and C.M., but he had to wait until he was twenty-one years of age, on April 19th 1893, before he could be admitted to the medical register. He took a job as locum tenens in a practice at Mere, Wiltshire, but when it was discovered that he could not sign a death certificate he was promptly dismissed. Soon after qualifying he did a short locum at Clydach Vale, Rhondda, and made the round voyage to Japan as a ship's surgeon. His first appointment was as assistant to Dr Frederick Heaton, an elderly G.P. who had an old established practice in the cathedral city of St Asaph. In 1896 at the age of twenty-four years he took the M.D. degree.

He had been three years at St Asaph when he saw an advertisement for a ' surgeon ' to the Park and Dare collieries at Cwmparc, Rhondda, in other words it advertised for a colliery doctor, who had to provide free medical attendance, free medicine and dressings for the miners and their families, for which the doctor was paid according to what was termed the ' poundage ' system, threepence in the pound being deducted from the miners' wages in order to pay the doctor for his services. Dr John was one of 144 applicants for the post, and the choice was made as a result of a ballot by the miners, and the final result was a victory for the ' young north Walian.' Dr John lived at Aeron Villa with his sister Elizabeth, who acted as his housekeeper. He soon built himself a large house which he named ' Gilnockie ', after an ancestral home of the Clan Armstrong. The life of a colliery doctor in the Rhondda was indeed hard. He attended three surgeries each day and on his daily rounds saw from thirty to seventy patients. Night calls were, more often than not, unnecessary, but no call was ever refused. Dr John, when his practice reached its peak maintained four surgeries and employed two doctors, two dispensers and a trained nurse. Since there was no dentist in the Rhondda, qualified or unqualified, Dr John extracted an average of six teeth each day, without any anaesthetic. Most of his emergency operations were carried out on the kitchen table, so he felt the need of a Cottage Hospital, but he had to wait until 1926 before Pentwyn Hospital was built. Among his many appointments was that of parish doctor and public vaccinator. At the time of the South African War he was commissioned as surgeon-captain in the local Volunteer Corps. Later he became brigade surgeon to the St John Ambulance Brigade.

In 1897 Dr John experienced an epidemic of diphtheria, which in those days had a very high mortality rate. In 1890 diphtheria anti-toxin was introduced so he had a new therapeutic weapon with which to combat the disease. A full account of his cases and his treatment was published in the *Lancet* in 1899 under the title, ' On the use of diphtheria antitoxin in general practice with the results of the treatment of 122 cases of diphtheria'. His object in publishing his paper was an endeavour to remove any lingering doubts of his fellow G.P.'s as to the efficacy of the treatment and its safety. Dr John died after a short illness, on December 29th 1931 after 35 years in practice. After his death the miners voted unanimously that Dr John's practice should fall into the capable hands of his brother, Fergus, whose practice at Ton-Pentre was adjacent to the Treorchy practice.

Dr Fergus Armstrong had had an excellent academic record. He received a secondary education at Abergele County School where his father was a governor, and from here he passed the London Matriculation examination, in the first class at the age of sixteen. In October 1904 he was registered as a medical student at Edinburgh University Medical School, and in 1909 he passed the final examination for the degree of M.B. Ch.B., at the age of twenty one, and he was registered as a general medical practitioner on August 6th 1909. He commenced his medical career as assistant to his brother John at Treorchy, at a salary of £150 per annum. Having spent a year at Treorchy he decided to study for a higher degree in medicine, and to apply for a post of house physician at Cardiff Royal Infirmary, in which he was successful. In 1912 he submitted a thesis for the M.D. (Edinburgh) on the subject, 'Creatinine as a test for malignant disease of the liver', which was highly commended by the examiners, and he passed the complete examination 'with honours'. He now turned his attention to a higher qualification in surgery, the diploma of F.R.C.S. Edinburgh. In October 1912 he went to Edinburgh with the object of studying for the fellowship. To keep himself, he obtained an appointment as supervisor of medical students in the department of anaesthetics. He had been the first to introduce the open ether method at the Cardiff Royal Infirmary and at the gynaecological wards of the Edinburgh Royal Infirmary. Dr Fergus has estimated that in his lifetime he gave some five thousand general anaesthetics without a death. He attended a coaching class in Edinburgh during the last quarter of 1912, and in January 1913 he passed the F.R.C.S. examination at the minimum age of twenty-five. He passed all his examinations in the shortest possible time and at the lowest possible age. He scorned all offers of a job commensurate with his qualifications and experience, which might have led to an appointment as consulting surgeon on the staff of the Cardiff Royal Infirmary, and instead he accepted a partnership in a colliery practice at Ton-Pentre, Rhondda, whose principal was Dr

Edward Hughes 'surgeon' to the Eastern and Maindy collieries, at a salary of £250 per annum. He commenced work as an assistant in January 1914, and only a few months later, on August 4th 1914, came the great upheaval caused by the outbreak of the First World War. He rushed to join the Forces, knowing that his patients would be well looked after by the principal, Dr Hughes, who had agreed to postpone his retirement until the war was over.

Dr Fergus was given a temporary (six months) commission as first lieutenant in the Royal Army Medical Corps. The Welsh Hospital was being formed at Netley at the time and he was sent to join that hospital as second in command with the rank of captain. After a few months he felt frustrated by the routine duties and yearned for the feel of a scalpel and the smell of the operating theatre. Having seen an advertisement which said, 'Wanted, Chief Surgeon to First British Hospital to Serbia, apply H. S. Souttar, Harley Street', off he went, and at the interview Mr Souttar told him, 'You are the man I want, you can have my place as I cannot go to Serbia'. Within a week of the six months commission having ended, he found himself on Good Friday 1915 on board ship bound for Salonika, which was reached on April 5th 1915. And now began his Odyssey through the Ruritanian countries of the Balkans. In company with Professor Strong of Harvard University, he travelled through Albania and Macedonia, over mountainous regions in order to inoculate some 30,000 troops, and on the way they found soldiers dying from malaria through lack of quinine.

On his return to his base, his contract with the First British Hospital having expired, he joined the Serbian Relief Fund's Hospital, whose commandant was Lady Leila Paget. The chief surgeon having been invalided out, Captain Armstrong was given his job. Here in its 1250 beds he gathered a wide and varied experience of war surgery. He carried on until October 21st 1915, when the Serbian Army having suffered a crushing defeat at the hands of the Austrian and Bulgarian armies was in retreat. The hospital and its staff surrendered and were taken prisoner. On March 1st 1916 the prisoners were taken over the mountains to Sofia, Bulgaria, where they were interned. At the end of a month they were moved across the Danube to Bucharest, Roumania, where they were liberated under the rules of the Geneva Convention. His own capture by the enemy had been dramatic. He was attending casualties in the operating theatre in the midst of a bombardment, when in walked a Bulgarian officer who said simply, in fluent English, ' You are my prisoner, 'adding that he was bringing in a badly wounded lieutenant, a colonel's son. Dr Fergus said that in this battle he worked continously for seventy-two hours without a break. After being in captivity for six months he was liberated in October 1916 and repatriated by the Red Cross after a long train journey which took him through the northern countries of Europe. As a duly appointed King's Messenger he delivered some thirty-two dispatch cases to our Foreign Office. While in Roumania he met Queen Marie of Roumania and worked in her hospital. He promised to return to work in her hospital if he was needed.

On his way to Treorchy he stayed for a week in London. As he was seeing a friend off at Euston Station he slipped and fell, injuring his ankle. X-rays showed a fracture. He was put in plaster and given crutches. He had hardly recovered from his injury when he received a telegram from Queen Marie which read, ' Come out at once to Palace, Bucharest ', and immediately he started making arrangements for his return to Roumania. In the meantime he was engaged in writing an article, entitled, ' War surgery in Serbia : penetrating wounds of the abdomen ', which was published in the *Lancet* in 1917. In October 1916 he set out on the long trek back to Roumania, and he took with him a team which included Dr Breckenridge Bayne, an American surgeon ; Sister O'Neill, his theatre sister while in Serbia and Ivan Campbell, an actor, whom Fergus had trained as an anaesthetist in the administration of open ether. When the Germans finally invaded Roumania, Dr Fergus and Sister O'Neill were advised to leave the country. In addition to escorting Miss O'Neill on the homeward journey, he looked after Miss Leila Milne, governess to the daughters of Queen Marie and formerly governess to the Connaught princesses.

When Queen Marie was recovering from an attack of appendicitis, she told Miss Milne that if an operation was necessary she would like Captain Armstrong to do it.

Before he finally left Roumania he developed a pustule on the dorsum of his right hand which was diagnosed by his friend Professor Jonescu, the famous Roumanian surgeon, as anthrax. He was treated by Sclavo's serum and cauterization, the scars of which can still be seen on his hand. When the party reached Stockholm they were invited to lunch with the Crown Prince and Princess of Sweden.

On the way home he took a trunkful of surgical instruments with him, but the customs officials at St Petersburgh refused to let it through the customs barrier. He was sent to see Trotsky, who, however, was equally adamant in his refusal. Nevertheless, he turned up at the station with his trunk, and after a long argument with an official who spoke English, he declared that the trunk contained the tools of his trade. This was enough for the official who promptly put a chalk mark on the trunk and let it past the barrier. The man refused a handsome tip saying, ' Bolsheviks never accept tips.'

He had returned home from the First World War with several decorations conferred upon him by the kings of Serbia and Roumania; from Serbia the Royal Red Cross of Serbia, and from Roumania the Order of Officer of the Star of Roumania, the country's highest decoration. He had the honour of being commissioned as a major in the Serbian Medical Corps. After his capture by the Bulgarians the enemy wanted to give him a medal for bravery, and they were very disappointed when it was pointed out that the British Government could not countenance the wearing of an enemy decoration in wartime. Lady Paget said that he had been recommended for a British decoration. but was deemed to be ineligible on account of his having been under the command of the Serbian army at the time.

Among his fellow-residents at the Cardiff Royal Infirmary he had been generally known as the ' Baron ', and some of them continued to address him by that title to the end of their days. When he wore the magnificent sable fur coat, which he had purchased in St Petersburgh, I must say that he looked ' every inch a baron '.

After his return home in February 1918 he took up the practice he had left so hurriedly in 1914. He well remembers the first emergency operation he performed when he joined the practice in Ton-Pentre. A woman aged eighty-five years was suffering from a strangulated hernia, and the operation was performed while the patient was lying on her own bed, in her own home. The patient was given a general anaesthetic which consisted of pure chloroform. In the middle of the operation the electric light failed and the operation was completed by candlelight. The patient made an uneventful recovery despite the candle droppings which found their way into the wound !

In a letter to the *British Medical Journal* in 1951 Dr Fergus said that between the years 1946 and 1951 he had performed five hundred appendicectomies without a death.

In the year 1930 he attended the annual meeting of the British Medical Association at Winnipeg, when he was thrilled to have the privilege of being shown round the famous Mayo Clinic and being able to talk to the brothers Charles and William Mayo.

For years he had been tormented by a duodenal ulcer, and in 1938 at the age of fifty-one he underwent the operation of gastro-enterostomy at Llandough Hospital. It was suggested that he needed a prolonged convalescence such as a world cruise could provide, so it was arranged that he should join the R.M.S. *Franconia,* as ship's surgeon, for a voyage round the world lasting five and a half months. The ship carried two doctors, the other being Dr Thoresby the permanent ship's surgeon. While on the high seas he performed an appendicectomy on a Bell Boy, aged fourteen. Dr Thoresby gave the anaesthetic and everything went like clockwork. The patient had a smooth and uninterrupted recovery.

Dr Fergus had been bombed and shelled during the First World War, but he had never been nearer to being a casualty than when the small mining village of Cwmparc was blitzed on the night of April 19th 1941. He was attending a patient in one of the little terraced houses when an inspector of police entered, and begged him to cross to the other side of the road to attend a more badly injured victim. No sooner had he left the house before a bomb fell on it, demolishing the house and killing its nine inhabitants. Twenty three persons lost their lives that night and many more were injured. Dr Fergus and his assistant dealt with all the casualties, except one who was transferred to the Cardiff Royal Infirmary, without having to call upon the Emergency Medical Service for assistance.

Of the nine surviving children of Charles and Janet Armstrong, four became doctors. Besides John and Fergus there were George William Armstrong, who went into general practice at Pontllanfraith, Monmouthshire, and Mrs Janet Herdman who became a school medical officer.

Dr Fergus was a generous host at 'Gilnockie' to the professional vocalists, musicians, actors, and adjudicators, who paid professional visits to the Rhondda. Among them over the years were such celebrities as Vic Oliver, Sir Adrian Boult, Sir Geraint Evans, and Eva Turner, to name only a few.

The writer has endeavoured to give a short biographical sketch of two remarkable brothers, doctors both, who had much in common ;

both took their final examinations at a very early age, and both spent the greater part of their professional lives in exacting and laborious colliery practice, where each acted as second opinion to the other since their practices were contiguous. Both remained bachelors, and indeed it could be said of them that they were married to their profession. Each will occupy an honoured place in the History of Medicine in Wales. When Dr Fergus retired, at the age of eighty, the local M.P. said, ' It is the end of a dynasty '. Now aged eighty seven, he is happily still with us.

I acknowledge with gratitude the help I have received from my wife and Dr John Lowe, among many others.

TWO AND A HALF CENTURIES OF MEDICAL PRACTICE
A WELSH MEDICAL DYNASTY

NIGEL NAUNTON DAVIES

This short paper is a highly personal one in that it concerns my own family and its forbears. There have been whimsical writings recently which have speculated on the possibility of medical families being genetically based. This account of one such medical dynasty tends to suggest that this is not likely as an explanation.

The family tree shows in abbreviated form the medical sections of the family and as far as practicable only those directly relevant to my title, omitting many in each generation who have not been medical, and many who have only intermarried with other medical families. For the most part the family has practised in the Rhondda Valleys.

The numbering of the family groups has, for convenience, started with my own group because it is the longest unbroken medical line for seven generations. In Group 3 there are breaks in the continuity in generations six and seven, but it resumes in generations eight and nine. The intermarriage with the descendants of the Rev. David Naunton in 1826 brought the Naunton name firmly into the tree throughout. The Naunton family is well documented, and in the fifteen generations before the Rev. David Naunton there are no traces of any medical leanings.

When the Rev. Henry Davies came to the valleys from Carmarthenshire, having been ordained there in 1718, they were wild, remote and beautiful wooded valleys, peopled by a very few of the highly independent hill farmers known as the *Gloran*. As far ahead as 1837, when the region was just being discovered by the outside world it was described by writers in ecstatic terms. ' There are few regions on earth that present more of the sublime and beautiful features of nature within the same compass than are to be found among the mountains, hills and valleys of the north of Glamorganshire '. Other phrases from their writings ' the salmon leaps . . . the wild river scenes . . . the emerald greenness . . . hardly surpassed through the alpine north . . .' make one realise how rapidly industry can destroy a region aesthetically.

As often happened in those times the Rev. Henry in his travels on horseback practised religion and medicine simultaneously. Unfortunately his notebooks have disappeared, but the book of extracts from them published after his death *Hen Lyfr Henry Davies* has recently come to light. His name is always quoted as being synonymous with the origins of Nonconformity in the Rhondda, and he founded the first chapel in the whole region at Cymmer, Porth in 1740—now sadly making way for a new by-pass road. He it was who brought Howell Harris, Trevecca, to the Rhondda, and his nauseatingly fervid correspondence with him as been preserved (*Y Cofiadur*).

In 1766 he fell from his horse into the river and was drowned. His son Samuel combined general practice with farming—in those days a common combination—and continued until he went blind. The second Henry, his son, had an extensive practice. Roads did not exist, the valleys were steep and wooded, and travel on horseback must have occupied a very great deal of his time. The population of the region only reached five hundred by 1801 and even these few people probably occupied him fully. As we know, he would probably have stayed with very ill people or they with him, as was the custom of the time.

His son, Evan, was a ' character '. His lifetime spans a period of vast change locally and nationally, in medicine and outside it, and saw the foundation of most of the associations and journals which are now still with us. He was energetic and wide-ranging in his interests, wrote extensively on theology as a keen Unitarian, and contributed to *Seren Gomer*, often under his bardic name of ' Ieuan ap Dewi '.

In 1827 he published at his own expense a duoglot magazine ' *The Family Doctor* ' (*Y Meddyg Teuluaidd*) with the Welsh and English side by side on the same page.

It anticipated by well over a century the B.M.A. publication of the same name, and must surely be one of the earliest examples of a medical question-and-answer column for the public. It ran for only four issues, presumably from lack of support.

The first coal was found in the Rhondda valleys, near their mouth in 1809, and Evan Davies was medical officer to the first colliery. Not until 1832 did industry penetrate up the valleys, but by 1855 there were twenty-seven pits and by 1914 about sixty-two. Now there are only two. In the ensuing 100 years the population multiplied three hundred times.

Conditions underground at that time were appalling, safety precautions non-existent, and the accidents constant. Evan Davies, as remained the custom in the coal industry until nationalisation, was paid by a compulsory deduction from the wages of the miners ('poundage'). There was no hospital and all injuries and operations had to be dealt with on the spot, in the home, or in the consulting room. Child labour, from the age of six, was normal, for twelve hours a day, usually underground, alone and in total darkness. The commonest occupation for children was opening and closing the underground doors for the trucks to pass.

Evan Davies married in 1826 Catherine Naunton, one of the six children of the Rev. David Naunton, who built (the roof with his own hands) the first Baptist Chapel in the valleys, called 'Nebo', at Ystradyfodwg. Before being ordained as a clergyman he was a road and pit contractor and was stated at the time to be the first tram line builder in Britain. Certainly he built the first tram line in the region, for the conveyance of coal, before any roads were built.

Three of Evan and Catherine's six children either died in infancy or were unmarried. The other three founded families (groups 1, 2 and 3) which are relevant here.

Group 1 started with my grandfather, Dr Idris Naunton Davies, the youngest. He too was a general practitioner, who was unusual in those days in marrying as a medical student. He married three times in all, his first two wives dying, and was survived for a further sixty-four years by his matriarchal widow, who died in 1953, aged nearly ninety-seven. When widowed she continued to own and run the practice with employed assistants for a considerable time.

My father, who qualified in 1910, worked for a time at the London Chest Hospital with the late Sir Thomas Lewis, and we used to have at home some of the original smoked drum tracings which Sir Thomas and he produced there; they remained firm friends and when University College Hospital Medical School was evacuated to Cardiff during the Second World War they took up the threads again. He was an assistant Medical Officer of Health in the Rhondda until the Great War, when he joined the R.A.M.C. When invalided out he worked for a while at the Ministry of Pensions, before joining a cousin (H.C.C. Joyce in Group 3) in general practice outside Cardiff. During his time in the Valleys he could count twenty-six of his relatives simultaneously in practice in the region.

I was briefly in partnership with him until he died in 1949, when I moved to my present practice in Kent, thus ending two hundred years of medical practice in Wales in direct lineage.

In Group 2 the late Idris Naunton Davies, with the same name as my grandfather, must be noted. After ten years in practice he decided to study for higher qualifications and whilst continuing in a busy industrial practice he became within two years M.D., M.R.C.P. and D.P.H. He then settled down for a further fifteen years in general practice before joining the Pneumoconiosis Research Unit of the Medical Research Council. One of his treasured appointments was High Constable of Miskin Higher, a rare and ancient office dating back twelve hundred years ! Evan and Catherine's eldest son, Henry Naunton Davies (founder of Group 3) was probably the most famous of the family in his lifetime. He was an impressive figure and left his mark. Born in 1827, and educated privately in Swansea he went to Guy's where he qualified in 1854, and then continued to take further examinations for the next nineteen years. He was a member of the old Provincial Medical and Surgical Association, and then was a founder member of the South Wales and Monmouthshire B.M.A., becoming president in 1887. He lived and practised in Porth for the whole of his life, where he became surgeon to eleven collieries and works, M.O.H., Certified Factory Surgeon, and Public Vaccinator. He helped to found Porth Cottage Hospital in 1894 and the plaque commemorating his contribution is still there. The ward named after him is now a surgical theatre suite. It is interesting to recall that for an industrial population of two hundred thousand the only previous hospital beds were the four at Tyntyla Cottage Hospital, founded seven years before. These four beds were bitterly opposed as being excessive ! He founded the Naunton Chapter of Royal Arch Freemasons, he was a J.P. and an Alderman for Glamorgan. A contemporary writer, the Rev. William Thomas 'Glanffrwd' wrote of him that he was 'a fine Welshman, fond of the language, literature, and the most experienced doctor in the country. His fame was widespread. If any relative of mine required a consultation on account of illness and I had permission to give my opinion I should whisper the name of

Dr Davies, Cymmer, in preference to any other doctor in the country.'

One of his interesting and well-known habits was to take elderly patients on visits to London, and thus to enjoy their enjoyment of a totally new world. The poundage system produced a good income and assistants were always employed and apparently readily available.

On 11th April, 1877, there occurred at Troedyrhiw Colliery, Cymmer, Porth, the disaster which has become known as the Tynewydd Colliery Disaster. It was a sudden inundation with immediate loss of life, some later during rescue attempts, and finally the astonishing rescue after ten days of four men and a boy. This involved cutting through forty yards of solid coal. The story of the rescue and the endless problems involved is a long and fascinating one and fortunately fully documented. Dr Henry Naunton Davies led the team of nine medical men who remained at the colliery for the whole ten days and nights.

At the B.M.A. Annual Meeting, at Manchester, in August of that year it was decided to institute the award of a Gold Medal for distinguished merit, and to award the first one to Dr Henry. The citation reads 'For heroic conduct, self-denial and humanity at a colliery disaster at Pontypridd.'

A Mansion House Fund was started by the Lord Mayor of London and because no professional men were eligible for the awards which were made to the rescuers, each was presented with an inscribed silver salver. The one presented to my grandfather was on display at this Congress exhibition. A large portrait of Dr Henry now hangs in the B.M.A. Welsh headquarters at Cardiff.

As a result of this disaster Queen Victoria was persuaded by public opinion to award the Albert Medal for heroism on land, as well as on the sea as originally stipulated. Twenty-five were awarded on this occasion.

In Group 4 Naunton Wingfield Davies, 1852-1925, was the first F.R.C.S. in the family. He was well known as a novelist and playwright, and one of his plays, 'The Cobweb', was subsequently filmed.

The last Group, 5, is remarkable for the sheer number of medical men, medical women and medical marriages in the Naunton Morgan family. The best known of the family is Sir Clifford Naunton Morgan, now retired from full-time surgical practice at Barts and St Marks, whose fame, particularly in his speciality, is widespread. His son,

Michael Naunton Morgan is a consulting surgeon to the Westminster Hospital.

I am sad that it is now official policy to discourage medical families. I make no apologies for my family and its contribution and I hope that it will continue here and there.

I believe that such families can contribute to the ethos of medicine.

BIBLIOGRAPHY

Alexander, D. T. (1915), *Glamorgan Reminiscences*. Spurrell, Carmarthen.

Barber, J. T. (1803). *A Tour through South Wales and Monmouthshire.* Cadell and Davies, London.

Cliffe, C. F. (1854). *The Book of South Wales*, 3rd ed. Hamilton, Adams, London.

Davies, E. N. (1846). *Rhifedi ac Undod Duw*. Cardiff.

Lloyd, J. E., Jenkins, R. T. and Sir W. L. Davies (1959). *Dictionary of Welsh Biography down to* 1940. Cymmrodorion Society, London.

Evans, R. M. (1972). *Children in the Mines:* 1840–42. National Museum of Wales, Cardiff.

"Glanffrwd" (William Thomas). (1949). *Llanwynno*. Gwasg Prifysgol Cymru, Caerdydd.

"Rufus" (J. R. Williams), (1864) *Hen Lyfr H. D.* (Henry Davies). Llangollen.

Hepburn, W. B. (1972). *Br. Med. J.* 1, 623.

Johns, D. B. (1910) *Early History of the Rhondda Valleys*. Pontypridd..

Lewis, E. D. (1959) *The Rhondda Valleys*. Phoenix House, London.

Lewis, E. & P. (1937). *The Land of Wales*. Batsford, London.

Malkin, B. H. (1807), *The Scenery, Antiquities & Biography of South Wales*, 2nd ed. London.

"Morien" (Owen Morgan) (1903). *History of Pontypridd and the Rhondda Valleys*. London.

Naunton Davies. J. The Tynewydd Mine Disaster of 1877. (Unpublished).

Owain, O. L. (1948), *Hanes y Ddrama yng Nghymru*, 1850–1943. H. Evans a'i Feibion, Liverpool.

Rees, T. (1815). *A Topographical and Historical Description of South Wales*. Sherwood, London.

Rees, T. M. (1908). *Notable Welshmen*. 'Herald' Office, Caernarvon.

Ap Rhys, M. (1938). *Eglwys Annibynnol y Cymer, Rhondda: Braslun o'i Hanes*, 1738–1938. D. J. Jones, Porth.

Roscoe, T. (1837). *Wanderings and Excursions in South Wales*. Tilt, Simpkin, London.

Trafodion Cymdeithas Hanes Bedyddwyr Cymru (1959, 1960 and 1964). Llandysul.

Williams, J. R. (1886) *Ystradiana*. Ystrad Rhondda.

Y Cofiadur. (1935). Wrexham.

LIST OF SPEAKERS

Dr Marshall W. Annear, Consultant Psychiatrist, Morgannwg Hospital.

*Dr D. J. B. Ashley, Consultant Pathologist, Morriston Hospital.

Dr John Cule, Lecturer in the History of Medicine, Welsh National School of Medicine.

Dr G. C. Davies, Senior House Officer (Surgery), Westminster Hospital.

Dr Howard E. F. Davies, Consultant in Geriatric Medicine, Gwent.

Dr John Davies, Lecturer, Department of Welsh History, University College of Wales, Aberystwyth.

Dr N. Naunton Davies, General Practitioner, Maidstone.

Dr Robert Gittings, Poet & Writer, Chichester.

Dr R. A. Griffiths, Senior Lecturer, Department of History, University College of Swansea.

Mr W. Gerallt Harries, Lecturer, Department of Welsh, University College of Swansea.

Dr Geoffrey A. Hodgson, Consultant Dermatologist, University Hospital of Wales.

Dr Arthur Hollman, Consultant Cardiologist, University College Hospital, London.

Dr D. Geraint James, Dean, Royal Northern Hospital, London.

Dr A. Trevor Jones, Past Provost, Welsh National School of Medicine.

Dr Emyr Wyn Jones, Consulting Cardiologist, Liverpool.

Dr Glyn Penrhyn Jones (decd.) Consultant Geriatrician, Caernarfon.

Dr Glynne Jones, Senior Registrar, University Hospital of Wales.

Baroness Lee of Asheridge opened the Conference with a paper on the contribution of Aneurin Bevan to the National Health Service.

Dr J. Gwynne Morgan, Retired, Clydach.

Dr Arthur Morris, Retired, Eastbourne.

Morfydd E. Owen, Lecturer, Department of Welsh, University College, Cardiff.

Dr E. Posner, Consultant Chest Physician, Stoke-on-Trent.

Dr K. Bryn Thomas, Consultant Anaesthetist, Royal Berkshire Hospital, Reading.

Dr Peter H. Thomas, Hon. Curator, Museum, Royal College of General Practitioners.

Dr Eirian Williams, Consultant Physician, Pembroke County Hospital, Haverfordwest.

*Paper—"Welshness" and Disease,—published in *Human Biology*, (1968), 40, pp. 517-533.

INDEX